The Science and Practice of Stuttering Treatment

A Symposium

T0256945

The Science and Practice of Stuttering Treatment

A Symposium

Edited by

Suzana Jelčić Jakšić

Speech pathologist, 'Sisters of Mercy' University Hospital Center, Children's Hospital, Zagreb, Croatia
President, Croatian Association for People Who Stutter 'Hinko Freund'
Director, Logopedski centar, Zagreb

Mark Onslow

Professor, Australian Stuttering Research Centre, University of Sydney, Sydney, Australia
Director, Australian Stuttering Research Centre

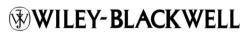

A John Wiley & Sons, Ltd., Publication

This edition first published 2012, © 2012 by John Wiley & Sons, Ltd.

Wiley-Blackwell is an imprint of John Wiley & Sons, formed by the merger of Wiley's global Scientific, Technical and Medical business with Blackwell Publishing.

Registered office: John Wiley & Sons, Ltd, The Atrium, Southern Gate, Chichester, West Sussex, PO19 8SQ, UK

Editorial offices: 9600 Garsington Road, Oxford, OX4 2DQ, UK
The Atrium, Southern Gate, Chichester, West Sussex, PO19 8SQ, UK
2121 State Avenue, Ames, Iowa 50014-8300, USA

For details of our global editorial offices, for customer services and for information about how to apply for permission to reuse the copyright material in this book please see our website at www.wiley.com/wiley-blackwell.

The right of the author to be identified as the author of this work has been asserted in accordance with the UK Copyright, Designs and Patents Act 1988.

Library of Congress Cataloging-in-Publication Data
The science and practice of stuttering treatment : a symposium / edited by Suzana Jelčić Jakšić and Mark Onslow.
     p.   cm.
   Includes bibliographical references and index.
   ISBN 978-0-470-67158-0 (pbk. : alk. paper)
   1. Stuttering–Treatment–Congresses.   2. Speech therapy–Congresses.
I. Jelčić Jakšić, Suzana.   II. Onslow, Mark.
   RC424.S384 2012
   616.85′54-dc23
                                                      2012005851

A catalogue record for this book is available from the British Library.

Wiley also publishes its books in a variety of electronic formats. Some content that appears in print may not be available in electronic books.

Cover image: © Shutterstock
Cover design: Sandra Heath
Stuttering logo by Likovni Studio, Ltd. Based in part on an Ancient Egyptian hieroglyphic thought to depict stuttering.

Set in 9/12.5 pt Interstate Light by Aptara® Inc., New Delhi, India
Printed in Singapore by Ho Printing Singapore Pte Ltd

1 2012

Contents

List of Contributors

Susan Block
La Trobe University
Melbourne, Australia

Michael Blomgren
The University of Utah
Salt Lake City, UT, USA

Elizabeth A. Cardell
University of Queensland
Brisbane, Australia

Brenda Carey
The University of Sydney
Sydney, Australia

Angela Cream
Osborne Park Hospital
Perth, Australia

Jason H. Davidow
Hofstra University
Hempstead, NY, USA

Francesca Del Gado
CRC Balbuzie
Rome, Italy

Rosemarie Hayhow
Speech & Language Therapy Research Unit
Bristol, UK

Sarita Koushik
University of Newcastle
Newcastle, Australia

and

Montreal Fluency Centre
Westmount, QC, Canada

Deborah Kully
Institute for Stuttering Treatment and Research
University of Alberta
Edmonton, AB, Canada

Marilyn Langevin
University of Alberta
Montreal, AB, Canada

Mirjana Lasan
Logopedski Centar
Zagreb, Croatia

Emanuela Lucchini
University of Rome, La Sapienza
Rome, Italy

Sue O'Brian
The University of Sydney
Sydney, Australia

Mark Onslow
The University of Sydney
Sydney, Australia

Dave Rowley
De Montfort University
Leicester, UK

Bruce Ryan
California State University, Long Beach
Long Beach, CA, USA

Tim Saltuklaroglu
University of Tennessee
Knoxville, TX, USA

Rosalee C. Shenker
Montreal Fluency Centre
Montreal, QC, Canada

Darinka Šoster
Institute for Psychological Disorders and Speech Pathology
Belgrade, Serbia

Maria Grazia Spinetti
CRC Balbuzie
Rome, Italy

Jelena Tadić
Institute for Psychological Disorders and Speech Pathology
Belgrade, Serbia

Donatella Tomaiuoli
University of Rome, La Sapienza
Rome, Italy

Natasha Trajkovski
The University of Sydney
Sydney, Australia

Preface

The notion of a symposium is attributable to the ancient Greeks. Scholars would gather for several days and share their knowledge while dining and drinking. In essence, that is what we all did during May 2010 at the Hotel Croatia in Cavtat on the Adriatic Coast, albeit departing from the Greek tradition in the customary modern way with a separation of the knowledge sharing and the dining and drinking. And, with very few exceptions, we managed to depart from the customary excesses and distractions typical of the ancient Greek Symposium.

Apart from the ancient Greeks who had the outstanding idea to do such a thing, our convening of the Croatia Symposium were inspired by the work of others. One of us read the early symposia during the early and middle years of the last century convened by the founders of our profession in the United States (The Stuttering Foundation, 2007; Van Riper, 1981) and became determined to organise such an event in Croatia.

For the rest of us, the distal origins of our symposium and the pages that follow were the 1980s during the reading of two volumes. The first of these was a text by Prins and Ingham (1983). This was a transcription of presentations by authorities of the day, followed by transcriptions of interactions between them and their audience. On behalf of groups who retired after each presentation to discuss its content, a series of discussion leaders engaged the speaker. A similar format appeared with an edition of Seminars in Speech and Language (Volume 6, Number 2). The vibrancy of those discussions soared from their pages. There was a record for the reader not only of what the authorities of the day thought about various topics to do with stuttering, but insights into the immediate responses to those thoughts by their peers.

As near as we can remember, the more recent origin of what follows was some time between 6-11 May 2007, at the Adriatic coastal town of Cavtat. That was during the 8th World Congress for People Who Stutter, held at the Hotel Croatia. Somehow, the idea of an international clinical symposium came up in conversation; a symposium where as many of the clinical authorities of our day would attend and air their views for the consideration of peers. On 12 May 2007, before departing Cavtat, we finalised our initial plans to go ahead with such a symposium.

After several years planning, a conference titled 'Stuttering: a Clinical Symposium' occurred during 22-26 May 2010 at the Hotel Croatia in Cavtat. We invited all the international clinical authorities of the day that we could bring to mind; those whose authority was research or clinically based. Very few of our invitations were declined.

We arranged for peer review of each presentation during the conference. Conference attendees were 'observers' and 'discussants'. The latter were three invited groups of around 10 researchers and clinicians who, under the direction of one of three discussion leaders, retired for half an hour after each presentation to consider the presented material and to generate some discussion questions. During that half-hour period, the Conference observers remained in the presentation room with the presenter and ourselves. During this period, we facilitated a discussion between the presenter and the observers. After a half hour, the discussion groups returned and the discussion leaders engaged the presenters in discussion, which was recorded for later transcription.

What follows is a record of those days in Cavtat. The book chapters record each presentation and the discussions that followed. Subsequent to the Conference, presenters wrote up their presentations in a formal manner, using the outline that they had been given: first, an overview of the treatment, then an outline of any theoretical origins of the treatment, followed by an overview of the demonstrated, empirical value of the treatment. Then, presentations concluded with an overview of the advantages and disadvantages of the treatment, and a general conclusion and projection of where the future for that treatment might lead.

Spoken language during scholarly discussion is a much different thing, we discovered, to the written language suitable for a publication such as this. Verbally, we found, it takes much longer to convey material than can be achieved with carefully edited text. The challenge for us, then, was to reduce the discussions to their essential features while retaining their content. Comparing the final product with the transcriptions, we think that we have succeeded.

Two of the presentations and subsequent discussions in the following pages did not occur at Cavtat, but in retrospect. These are the contributions by Dr Jason Davidow and Dr Bruce Ryan, who accepted invitations to the Conference but were ultimately unable to attend. Those presenters submitted and finalised their chapters with us, and then we distributed them to the discussion leaders, who engaged those two presenters in an online discussion to produce the final product presented here. The book bears the inspirational title provided by our publishers, 'The Science and Practice of Stuttering Treatment: A Symposium'.

We did impose some ground rules for our authors about citations of scholarly work in support of their chapters. Citations were accepted only if they were to sources that would be reasonably available to the readership, such as other texts, journal articles and published conference proceedings. Citations of unpublished sources were allowed only to indicate the existence of some completed research or research in progress, but not to any of its results. When we made an exception to this rule we recorded the occurrence with a footnote. Authors were permitted to refer to unpublished treatment manuals, provided they made such manuals available to the readership by email and provided an email address in a footnote.

Under the heading 'Demonstrated Value', authors naturally overviewed any published data about the treatments they discussed. In such cases, we chose what we thought was the most compelling data in support of the treatment, and presented it in a simple graphical format. We made authors feel free to publish previously unpublished data in this section, and several of them took that option. We need to note, however, that in those cases the data presented are not peer reviewed in any sense of the term and should not be regarded by the readership as such.

For the sake of simplicity, we encouraged authors to use the term 'speech restructuring' throughout this text to refer to a generic style of speech treatment for stuttering control that includes variants known as 'prolonged speech', 'prolongation', 'smooth speech', 'passive airflow' and 'fluency shaping'. We use the following definition of speech restructuring, which in our view parsimoniously captures the essence of these treatments: 'a new speech pattern to reduce or eliminate stuttering while sounding as natural as possible' (Onslow and Menzies, 2010).

No symposium can happen on its own. We are indebted to support from various institutions for the Symposium: The University of Sydney, The Children's Hospital Zagreb and the Ministry of Science, Education and Sports of the Republic of Croatia.

We need to finish by registering our gratitude to people without whom this venture simply could not have occurred. Dave Rowley helped us with his professional lifetime of experience with organising the Oxford Dysfluency Conference. We don't know how we could have done things without him. So much so that, buoyed by the success of our first such venture, we thought we would do it all again in three years, and we plan to repeat the event every three years subsequently. We asked Dave to join us as a convenor of that future event, and we are delighted that he agreed to do so.

We are grateful for support and help from Mirjana Lasan during the local planning of the symposium. We also thank Danko Jakšić for his miraculous graphic skills that established a visual identity for symposium incorporating the Adriatic coast. In particular, he created the graphic that appears on the cover of this book, which we hope will be an enduring symbol of this event during future years.

The day to day logistics of the symposium would have been impossible if not for the professional and dedicated contributions made by students from the University of Zagreb: Lucija Božajić, Lea Horvat, Marija Kordić, Nina Kupusović, Maja Mrkajić and Ana Viđak. Those students made the logistics happen without failure of any kind. The success of the symposium depended ultimately on discussion groups leaving the conference room promptly, convening and considering their material in an efficient manner at another location, and returning to the conference room on time after half an hour. Most importantly, this book would not have been possible without clear audio recordings of the discussion leaders and the presenters for transcription. Those students made that happen. Our transcriptionist, Rosemary Cartwright, would not have been able to do her work effectively without this material.

It may not be obvious when reading the pages that follow, but the success of the symposium was due considerably to the talents of the discussion leaders: Ann Packman, Joe Attanasio and Sheena Reilly. Their quick-wittedness, as they rapidly collated probing discussion topics, their articulateness on the floor during discussion and their thoroughness as scientists and scholars left us bewildered. We can't think of any three people who could have done a better job.

There are two final people who warrant special mention. Somehow, we don't know how, Jasmine Katakos managed to provide financial management of the symposium and to make it a financial success. Again, we don't know how, but Victoria Brown patiently and effectively provided scientific copy editing of our crude attempts at assembling this text, without becoming particularly close to a nervous breakdown. Somehow, Jasmine and Victoria managed these feats in addition to their standard duties at the Australian Stuttering Research Centre. But had they not done so, we would never have found ourselves in Cavtat to enjoy such a wonderful experience, and we would never have been as proud as we are of this book that emerged from it all.

Suzana Jelčić Jakšić
Zagreb

Mark Onslow
Sydney
October 2011

References

Onslow, M., & Menzies, R. (2010) *Speech restructuring.* Accepted entry in www.commonlanguagepsychotherapy.org

Prins, D., & Ingham, R. (1983) *Treatment of stuttering in early childhood: Methods and Issues.* San Diego, CA: College-Hill Press.

The Stuttering Foundation (2007) Special anniversary newsletter: 60 years of service. The Stuttering Foundation.

Van Riper, C. (1981) An early history of ASHA. *ASHA Magazine, 23*(11), 855-858.

Chapter 1
Modifying Phonation Interval Stuttering Treatment Program

Jason H. Davidow

Hofstra University, Hempstead, NY, USA

Overview

Modification of phonation intervals

The Modifying Phonation Interval (MPI) Stuttering Treatment Program is a computer-aided, biofeedback programme based on reducing the occurrence of short intervals of phonation during speech production. Clients proceed through a series of performance-contingent steps, requiring the completion of several speech tasks in various situations. The goal of the programme is self-managed, stutter-free, natural-sounding and effortless speech in beyond-clinic settings. The MPI programme is intended for adults, adolescents and school-age children.

A phonation interval (PI) is a measure of the duration of vibration measured from the surface of the throat (via an accelerometer) in between breaks of 10 milliseconds (ms) or more. PIs are collected via the MPI system (Ingham et al., 2007), which runs in a Windows environment and consists of an accelerometer, a signal conditioning system, computer software and related hardware (see Davidow et al., 2009 for technical details). The software allows for the recording of all PIs and allows for PIs within a specified ms range (e.g. 30-120 ms) to be fed back (audio-visually) to the client in real time. Perceptually based measures of percent syllables stuttered (%SS), syllables per minute (SPM), speech naturalness (1-9 scale; 1 = highly natural, 9 = highly unnatural; Martin et al., 1984) and speech effort (1-9 scale; 1 = highly effortless, 9 = highly effortful) can also be gathered using the MPI software. Speech effort targets, however, are not part of the MPI treatment protocol outlined by Ingham et al. (2007).[1]

---

[1]Although not outlined in the Ingham et al. (2007) treatment manual, speech effort targets are part of the performance-contingent requirements in the currently used MPI treatment protocol. See Ingham, Ingham, and Bothe (in press) for a discussion regarding the use of speech effort ratings during treatment.

The Science and Practice of Stuttering Treatment: A Symposium, First Edition. Edited by Suzana Jelčić Jakšić and Mark Onslow.
© 2012 John Wiley & Sons, Ltd. Published 2012 by John Wiley & Sons, Ltd.

Pre-establishment

The MPI programme includes Pre-establishment, Establishment, Transfer and Maintenance Phases. The purpose of the Pre-establishment Phase is to collect baseline %SS, SPM and speech naturalness data, and to find the PI range that the client will manipulate (called the Functional or Target PI Range). The Target PI Range is found via several steps. First, the MPI software collects all of the client's PIs across 3-minute speaking tasks repeated on at least three occasions over the 2–3 month Pre-establishment Phase. PIs during normal speaking situations (reading, monologue, conversation) typically range from 10 to 1000 ms (very few PIs are longer than 1000 ms); however, PIs below 30 ms are discarded since they have been found to be too difficult to control and may be confounded by head and neck movements. Second, the software categorises the PIs into quintiles; that is, the software identifies the ms PI range that contains the lowest 20% of PIs (e.g. 30–60 ms PIs), the lowest 40% of PIs (e.g. 30–150 ms PIs), the lowest 60% of PIs (e.g. 30–290 ms PIs), and so on. Third, the client attempts to reduce the number of PIs by 50% in the lowest quintile range, which is now the Target PI Range, and tries to exert control of Target Range PIs (produce them on demand and produce longer PIs on demand) across several speaking tasks. If the client can accomplish this, the lowest 20% is used as the Target PI Range for the remainder of the treatment programme. If control is not shown over the 20% quintile range, the Target PI Range is increased in 10% increments (lowest 30%, then lowest 40%) until the client can reduce the number of PIs by 50% and exert control of them. The creators of the programme state that no participant has needed to go beyond the 40% quintile range to exert control (Ingham et al., 2007). No speaking style or speech rate is prescribed during this process; that is, the speaker needs to discover how to control PIs.

Establishment

The remaining phases of the programme are designed as performance-contingent schedules. The Establishment Phase consists of a series of speaking tasks of different lengths of time (see Ingham, 1999 for the complete treatment schedule), progressing from reading tasks to conversational tasks. Each speaking situation requires 1-minute, 2-minute and 3-minute trials. A trial is 'passed' if there is zero self-judged stuttering, self-judged naturalness of below 3 and target PIs are reduced by 50%. If these criteria are not met, the client repeats the trial or regresses in the treatment schedule. Additionally, the clinician judges the final speaking trial for each speaking situation and the criteria just mentioned must be met for progression to the next speaking situation. Clients are encouraged to attend daily 2–3 hour sessions within the clinic, but clients completing bi-daily sessions have had success with the programme (Ingham et al., 2007).

Transfer

The Transfer Phase, initiated at the completion of the Establishment Phase, includes several 3-minute beyond-clinic speaking tasks selected to reflect situations in the client's natural environment that are important to the client. Six different situations are required with three 3-minute trials passed for each situation. This results in eighteen 3-minute trials that must be passed. The progression includes telephone conversation, general conversation and self-selected tasks. A trial is 'passed' if it is judged stutter free and natural sounding (below 3 on the 1–9 scale) by the client, with the last trial for each task judged by the clinician. If these criteria are not met, the client repeats the trial or regresses in the treatment schedule.

Maintenance

The final phase, the Maintenance Phase, involves increased time between clinical visits as the reward for meeting 'pass' criteria. Three 3-minute speaking tasks are completed, and two of the tasks are scored and must be judged as stutter free and natural sounding by the client, while one is scored and must be judged as stutter free and natural sounding by the clinician. The duration of the Maintenance Phase in the current MPI manual (Ingham et al., 2007) is 22 weeks if no step is 'failed'. If any step is 'failed', the client returns to the beginning of the Maintenance Phase.

Theoretical basis

Research into PIs began as an empirically grounded search to operationalise the characteristics of prolonged speech (Ingham et al., 1983); see Preface for a definition of this term. Previous literature had shown that stutter-free speech was accompanied by increases in phonation time during delayed auditory feedback/prolonged speech (Goldiamond, 1965, 1967), in addition to other so-called fluency-inducing conditions (FICs), such as singing (Colcord and Adams, 1979) and chorus reading (Adams and Ramig, 1980), as researchers examined Wingate's 'Modified Vocalization Hypothesis' (Wingate, 1969, 1970). However, the effect on stuttering of directly manipulating any specific element of phonation time had not been studied.

Along with the idea that increased phonation time can decrease stuttering, two studies provided the initial motivation for focusing on reducing the occurrence of short PIs, rather than directly extending phonation. The first was a study by Adams and Hayden (1976) showing that adults who stutter had slower laryngeal reaction times than normally fluent controls. Although there were some findings to the contrary, the majority of subsequent studies confirmed this initial finding (see Bloodstein and Ratner, 2008, Chapter 5 for a review). The other study by Manning and Coufal (1976) provided 'additional evidence that stuttering is increased during speech that requires the rapid alternation of phonated and non-phonated sounds' (Ingham et al., 2001, p. 1229). These findings taken together compelled Gow and Ingham (1992) to conclude, '... it should follow that training to control the frequency of short intervals of phonation (presumably they require faster and more frequent initiation/termination of phonation) should control the frequency of stuttering ...' (p. 495).

The early PI studies were single-subject investigations (Gow and Ingham, 1992; Ingham and Devan, 1987; Ingham et al., 1983) validating the use of reducing the frequency of short PIs as a stuttering reduction agent. When participants reduced the frequency of short PIs (30–200 ms) in their speech by 50%, stuttering was reduced to zero or near-zero levels. In addition, when people who stutter (PWS) increased the number of short PIs in their speech back to baseline or above baseline levels, stuttering returned, although this was not a consistent finding (Gow and Ingham, 1992). In general, however, these studies showed that manipulating short PIs could control stuttering frequency. Speakers were also able to reduce the number of short PIs (accompanied by stuttering reductions) while receiving naturalness ratings between 3 and 6 on the 1–9 naturalness scale (Martin et al., 1984) using normal speaking rates. These latter findings revealed that attaining another goal of the MPI research line was possible, which was overcoming the problem of unnatural-sounding speech following speech-pattern style treatments such as prolonged speech that involved directly increasing phonation time.

Research into PIs was also motivated by a need to find a replicable procedure for manipulating phonation time (Ingham et al., 1983). The use of a computer and accompanying hardware to measure PIs was important for this purpose. Most prolonged speech programmes require perceptual judgment of task compliance by clinicians, a task that clinicians do with questionable reliability (Onslow and O'Brian, 1998). An objective measurement of the treatment target could aid in this difficult task and provide a more controlled way to modify stuttering. The early PI studies showed that participants could replicate the speech pattern and maintain stuttering reductions (Gow and Ingham, 1992; Ingham et al., 1983). In summary, the results of these early studies provided evidence for a desirable treatment outcome: a replicable speech pattern that produces stutter-free and natural-sounding speech, within normal speaking rates.

Demonstrated value

Besides the early PI studies that showed manipulating the number of short PIs resulted in changes in stuttering frequency (Gow and Ingham, 1992; Ingham and Devan, 1987; Ingham et al., 1983), several other pieces of literature provide support for the MPI treatment programme. First, and the most complete assessment of the MPI programme, was a long-term study by Ingham et al. (2001). In that study, five men who stutter ranging in age from 18 to 28 years demonstrated zero or near-zero stuttering during within- and beyond-clinic speaking contexts, 1 year into the Maintenance Phase. Their speech was also natural sounding and speaking rates increased. Figure 1.1 shows part of the results for this study from assessments when participants were speaking in the clinic and beyond the clinic on the telephone. These assessments were conducted without feedback from the MPI programme.

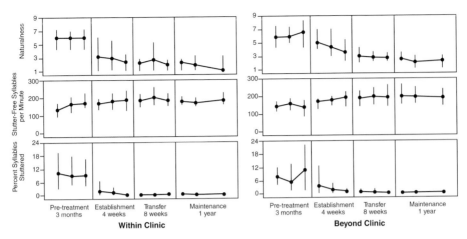

Figure 1.1 Means of assessments during within and beyond the clinic speaking situations for the five participants in the Ingham et al. (2001) report. The left panel shows results for telephone conversations and the right panel for self-selected speaking tasks. Speech naturalness scores, speech rate scores in stutter-free syllables per minute and stuttering rate in percent syllables stuttered are presented. The vertical bars represent the ranges for the five participants. Adapted by permission of the American Speech-Language-Hearing Association.

Second, in a positron emission tomography study, Ingham et al. (2003) found that a group of 17 participants who completed approximately half of the Establishment Phase exhibited normalised cerebral blood blow in brain regions that appear critical for fluency during a monologue task. Third, Davidow et al. (2009) found a reduction in the occurrence of short PIs (30–150 ms) during singing, chorus reading, prolonged speech and syllable-based metronomic speech. Packman et al. (1994) previously found a reduction in the 50–150-ms range during prolonged speech. Findings from these latter two studies suggest that a reduction in the number of short PIs may be influential in our understanding of the fluency-inducing mechanisms underlying the most powerful fluency-enhancing conditions (FICs), and they provide further support for the association between reducing the number of short PIs and stuttering reductions.

In addition to the value of the specific treatment technique (reducing the frequency of short PIs), many elements of the MPI treatment framework have substantial support in the literature. In the most recent comprehensive review of the stuttering treatment literature, Bothe et al. (2006) found that the most successful (largest reductions in stuttering and social, emotional and cognitive symptoms) treatments for adults who stutter are 'prolonged speech-type' treatments that include 'self-evaluation of speech and/or self-management of program steps, a focus on speech naturalness and feedback of naturalness measurements, and an active contingent maintenance program that continues to address not only stuttering but also speech naturalness and self-evaluation skills' (p. 335). The MPI programme includes all of these elements. The most successful treatments for school-age children and adolescents in the Bothe et al. review also included many of these treatment elements.

Advantages and disadvantages

Advantages

One of the unique advantages of the MPI programme is that the MPI system allows for an objective evaluation of the target speech pattern. This ensures maintenance of a speech pattern that has been found to induce fluency and eliminates the need for a subjective evaluation by a clinician. Although the necessity of accurate feedback of prolonged speech targets during treatment has not been established, more objective and reliable feedback of the target speech pattern may increase programme effectiveness (Onslow and O'Brian, 1998), particularly if the specific speech pattern manipulation has been shown to be important for reducing stuttering. Clients can also connect the MPI system to their home computer, which allows them to assess the targeted speech pattern at their convenience. Another advantage of the MPI programme, and one mentioned by MPI clients, is that emphasis on self-management provides the client with control during the treatment process (Ingham et al., 2001). Clients choose the time and duration of practice sessions, type of transfer tasks and evaluation situations during the Maintenance Phase. Other advantages include natural-sounding speech early in the treatment process, experimentally supported treatment procedures (see Section Demonstrated value), including evidence for increased probability of maintaining stuttering reductions using a self-managed, performance-contingent maintenance schedule (Ingham, 1980, 1982), and a step-by-step account of the treatment protocol (Ingham, 1999; Ingham et al., 2007), which eliminates guesswork by the clinician and the need for development of a highly individualised programme for each client.

Disadvantages

There are several issues with the MPI programme that require further inquiry. First, there is a lack of published, long-term follow-up data. To date, there is evidence from only five participants 1 year into the Maintenance Phase. Ingham et al. (2001) do state that 'all participants were also assessed in all beyond-clinic speaking conditions 12 months after the completion of the Maintenance Phase and showed levels of performance that were essentially identical to the levels reported at the completion of that phase' (p. 1241), but no data are provided. Second, the exact percentage of PIs to reduce within the Target PI Range, and the Target PI Range itself, require further study. The 50% reduction in the number of short PIs used to reduce stuttering was chosen initially for a series of unspecified reasons. Interestingly, however, the Davidow et al. (2009) study found percentage reductions in short PIs close to this value during several FICs. Similarly, although the lowest quintile range has been successful in reducing stuttering, a different range may be more advantageous. For example, the Davidow et al. study also found that PIs in the 51-150 ms range had the largest reduction. The lowest quintile range often extends past 150 ms. It may be more beneficial to just focus on the 51-150-ms range. Lastly, as mentioned by Ingham et al. (2001), determining the efficacy of the treatment package is important. In the Ingham et al. study, participants had unlimited access to the MPI system; that is, participants were allowed to practice with the MPI system outside of the treatment schedule throughout all of the treatment phases. Therefore, it is difficult to determine the necessity of this extra practice on the final treatment outcome and the efficacy of the complete treatment schedule or certain treatment phases as outlined in the MPI manual.

Conclusions and future directions

There are several conclusions that can be drawn from the MPI research line. First, reducing the number of short PIs can be a powerful fluency inducer for PWS. Second, in combination with a self-managed, performance-contingent treatment schedule, reducing the number of short PIs can result in long-term stutter-free, natural-sounding speech within normal speaking rates (Ingham et al., 2001). Lastly, further investigation into the role of PIs in reducing stuttering should continue, especially the collection and publication of long-term follow-up data after the completion of the Maintenance Phase. The results of the initial treatment study (Ingham et al., 2001) were promising and strongly suggest the value of a clinical trial with a larger, more varied group of participants.

Future PI research may include clarifying the issues in the immediately preceding section: percentage of short PIs to reduce, Target PI Range and efficacy of particular parts of the treatment package. More long-term outcome data should be obtained due to the recent opening of an MPI clinic at The University of California at Santa Barbara (UCSB, 2010). We are also currently exploring the necessity of PI alterations during FICs. Previous PI investigations have found reductions in the occurrence of short PIs during such conditions (Davidow et al., 2009; Packman et al., 1994); however, the necessity of these adjustments for fluency during the FICs has not been established. In order to determine this necessity, we are having speakers perform chorus reading and metronomic speech while attempting to not make the adjustment. Studies exploring the relationship of PI control to neural regions that might be functionally related to stuttering may also be conducted.

Acknowledgement

Special thanks are due to Roger Ingham for his assistance during the preparation of this chapter.

Discussion

Joseph Attanasio

You are rightly concerned about the reliability of perceptual or subjective clinician-provided feedback in prolonged speech programmes. Could you make a more compelling case, than you do in your presentation, in favour of the MPI Stuttering Treatment Program as an alternative to prolonged speech programmes; is your approach more effective in providing feedback than what is done in those other programmes? Is your programme more efficient than programmes that do not require the use of a computer?

Jason Davidow

Could you please clarify what you mean by 'more effective in providing feedback'? Do you mean accuracy, ability of the client to take the feedback and adjust the speech pattern, etc.?

Joseph Attanasio

Yes, exactly. You state that most prolonged speech programmes require clinicians to make perceptual judgments of task compliance but that they do so with questionable reliability. You also state that the necessity of accurate feedback of prolonged speech targets during treatment has not been established but, nevertheless, more objective and reliable feedback of the target speech pattern may increase programme effectiveness.

Jason Davidow

The effectiveness and efficiency of the computer-aided parts of the MPI programme over similar parts of prolonged speech treatments that are not computer-aided is an issue for future research. Direct comparisons of the MPI treatment study to other treatment literature are difficult, due to various methodological differences between the studies. For this reason, there are no direct comparisons in our presentation. The main advantage of a computer-aided programme over one relying on clinician feedback is likely to be that a clinician is not needed to reinforce correct production of the target speech pattern. This may allow for fewer clinician contact hours, possibly reducing the cost of therapy, particularly during the learning of the speech pattern. A client may also be more confident with performing the targeted speech pattern properly during beyond-clinic or maintenance exercises when using systems, like the MPI system, that can be connected to a home computer. This could reduce the need for 'refresher sessions' with a clinician during the Maintenance Phase of treatment.

Joseph Attanasio

My next question is somewhat related to what you state in your response. From your description of the programme, I take it that clients in the Transfer and Maintenance Phases do not necessarily use the computer. If I am correct, then in the absence of computer-assisted feedback, what do you think is operating to enable the client to produce stutter-free, natural-sounding speech? That is, can you be certain that there is a relationship between successful target PI reduction during the Establishment Phase of the programme and performance during the Transfer and Maintenance Phases?

Jason Davidow

Your question seems applicable to all treatments, not just computer-assisted treatments. Activities may be performed outside of the treatment protocol during transfer and maintenance that assist the client in retaining treatment benefits. The impact of those activities, or an influence such as maturation, on treatment outcome and their interaction with the treatment target would certainly provide valuable information for all stuttering treatments. That being said, the Ingham et al. (2001) report states that the participants performed 'periodic practice with the MPI system' (p. 1241) throughout the Transfer and Maintenance Phases, and an assessment during the Maintenance Phase showed that the participants maintained reductions in the number of short PIs from pre-treatment assessments, accompanied by zero or near-zero stuttering. If we assume, however, that an MPI client does not use the computer-assisted feedback during the Transfer and Maintenance Phases, there are several other components that could contribute to the maintenance of stutter-free and natural-sounding speech, including retaining the alteration in speech pattern that occurred during the Establishment Phase, the performance-contingent maintenance schedule, the focus on self-management, and the emphasis on beyond-clinic speaking tasks.

Joseph Attanasio

Thank you for that thoughtful and detailed response. Have you found that zero self-judged stuttering and self-judged naturalness below 3 can occur when the target PIs are not reduced by 50%?

Jason Davidow

The Ingham et al. (2001) study includes assessments during the Establishment and Maintenance Phases showing that some participants, although they were very close to it, did not quite reach the 50% reduction mark on certain occasions and still had zero stuttering (counted by raters). Unfortunately, I do not have access to the data needed to appropriately answer your question in regards to self-judged naturalness.

Ann Packman

We were wondering how the PI information is fed back audio-visually. Could you please explain?

Jason Davidow

The PIs are recorded and fed back to the speaker via a computer screen and brief tone. The software allows the user to specify a Target Range (e.g. 30–150 ms) and a dot is placed in the 'Target Range' box on the computer screen each time a PI in the Target Range is produced. There is also a brief tone as each dot appears.

Ann Packman

It seems that the Ingham et al. (2007) publication is the treatment manual. Is this available?

Jason Davidow

The current treatment manual is not available online. However, it is similar to the procedures outlined in the Ingham (1999) chapter. That chapter includes explanations of the Pre-establishment, Establishment, Transfer and Maintenance Phases, and a step-by-step description of the speaking tasks in each phase.

Ann Packman

The first report of the programme was in 2001 but the software is still not available for others to use. Can you estimate when it will be made available?

Jason Davidow

It will be available after the current long-term study is completed and the data for that study will continue to come in until next year. Some of those data were presented at a recent ASHA conference.

Ann Packman

Do you have some idea of which clients respond better to the programme? For example, do people with mild stuttering do better, or progress quicker?

Jason Davidow

I will answer that question using the data presented in the Ingham et al. (2001) study, since I do not have access to the relevant data from other clients using the MPI programme. As can be seen in the Ingham et al. study, the MPI treatment programme has been shown to be effective for clients with varying levels of stuttering. Stuttering frequency ranged from 4%SS to approximately 20%SS before treatment in that investigation. The information presented in the Ingham et al. study does not allow for determining the association between pre-treatment stuttering levels and time to progress through the programme. However, Figure 4 in that publication reveals the average time to complete each phase of the programme. That figure shows an average of 4 weeks to complete the Establishment Phase, 8 weeks for the Transfer Phase and 1 year for the Maintenance Phase.

Ann Packman

Is it possible to estimate how many clinician hours are required to conduct the programme?

Jason Davidow

The MPI programme has mainly been run in a research mode, so it is difficult to determine how many hours it will take to conduct the programme outside of a research context or the average number of face-to-face clinician hours needed to run the programme. Additional hours were needed to complete the components of the experimental protocols used during the MPI studies that would not be necessary in a clinical environment. However, the MPI clinic at UCSB was opened this past summer and the programme has been conducted in a non-research context with three clients in that clinic, allowing us a preliminary look at the number of face-to-face hours needed. The following is the current breakdown for clinician face-to-face time for these three clients for the routine MPI programme: 2.5 hours for pre-treatment assessment, 20–25 hours for the Establishment Phase, 3 hours for the Transfer Phase and 3 hours for the Maintenance Phase.

Sheena Reilly

My question concerns the applicability of the MPI programme for adults, adolescents and school-age children. What evidence is there to support using MPI for each of the age groups? I think the data referred to in the paper mainly concerns adults older than 18 years. Could you clarify and also explain why it would not be applicable for preschool-age children and is the programme delivered in exactly the same way for adults as for school-age children?

Jason Davidow

Yes, the data in the Ingham et al. (2001) study are from PWS, aged 18–28 years. As far as I know, there are no published treatment data for PWS under 18 years old. However, Ingham (1999) states that the programme has been conducted with adults and adolescents, and there are data for PWS under 18 years old in the experimental studies conducted during the development of the programme (Ingham and Devan, 1987; Ingham et al., 1983). The participants under 18 years old in those studies were able to reduce the frequency of short PIs in their speech with accompanying reductions in stuttering. I am unsure if the programme has been administered to school-age children. Perhaps the publication of the current long-term MPI study will include PWS under 18 years old.

Sheena Reilly

And preschool-age children?

Jason Davidow

As far as I know, the programme has not been conducted with preschool-age children. Although I can't speak to why the developers of the programme may not have run the programme with this age group, I can provide some of the reasons why I think the programme may not be applicable or a most appropriate option at this point in time as it is currently constructed. First, there are other programmes, such as the Lidcombe Program (LP), that seem more applicable. The LP has a solid research base with preschoolers and doesn't involve the issue of shaping the learned speech pattern into a natural-sounding pattern. Second, the MPI treatment schedule is somewhat intensive and often requires concentration over an extended period of time. It would probably be very difficult for a preschooler to focus on the necessary tasks for a long time. Third, the developers of the programme have structured the MPI programme so that it can be self-managed. It would likely be very difficult for a preschooler to manage several of these elements. A parent could possibly manage some of them, but others, including the reduction in the number of short phonated intervals that has to be understood by the client, would probably be too involved for a preschooler.

Sheena Reilly

This question concerns the dose and duration of the MPI programme. In the Establishment Phase the client is encouraged to attend 2–3 hour daily sessions.

Could you clarify how long these daily sessions are required and how long each of the three phases takes to complete. It would be good to know what the average time is and the range as well. Perhaps you could also comment on how feasible it is to transfer this to the 'real world'?

Jason Davidow

Using the text from the Ingham et al. (2001) treatment study, we can get a general idea of how many hours the Establishment Phase took for participants in that study. The authors state that this phase took about 2–3 weeks, using daily or bi-daily sessions of 2–3 hours. So, we can get an idea of the length of this phase by using the average of those values and calculating the number of hours for someone who performed the treatment daily, and someone who only performed the treatment schedule bi-daily (once every 2 days). If someone took 2.5 weeks (17.5 days) to complete this phase and came in once per day for 2.5 hours, the Establishment Phase would have been around 44 hours (17.5 days × 2.5 hours). If someone took 2.5 weeks (17.5 days) to complete this phase and came in every 2 days for 2.5 hours, the Establishment Phase would have been around 22 hours (8.75 days × 2.5 hours). It would seem that the average number of hours was probably somewhere between the two values of 22 and 44 hours. It should be noted that these are the hour values assuming that participants came in on the weekends, which may not have been the case. If the participants only came in during the week, the averages would be around 31 hours (daily) and 16 hours (bi-daily).

Ingham et al. (2001) state that the Transfer Phase took an average of 8 weeks to complete. The Transfer Phase would require 54 minutes of speaking if the client passed each of the speaking tasks on the first attempt. If every task was not passed on the first attempt, the amount of speaking time would vary depending on how many times the client did not meet the required criteria (stutter-free and natural-sounding speech). Ingham et al. also state that participants in that study were allowed to practice with the MPI programme during the Transfer Phase, and that an average of approximately 25 minutes of practice was completed per week. The Maintenance Phase would require 63 minutes of speaking if the client passed each of the speaking tasks on the first attempt. As with the Transfer Phase, if all tasks were not passed on the first attempt, the amount of speaking time in the Maintenance Phase would vary depending on how many times the criteria were not met.

Sheena Reilly

Could you comment on how use of this device in clinical trials would translate to clinical communities, the so-called real world.

Jason Davidow

An MPI clinic has been opened at UCSB in order to examine the effectiveness of the programme in a clinical context. It is still fairly early in the development of the MPI treatment, so it is not surprising that there are no published data, to the best of my knowledge, from Phase IV, or translational research.

References

Adams, M. R., & Hayden, P. (1976) The ability of stutterers and nonstutterers to initiate and terminate phonation during production of an isolated vowel. *Journal of Speech and Hearing Research, 19,* 290-296.

Bloodstein, O., & Ratner, N. B. (2008) *A Handbook on Stuttering* (6th ed.). New York: Thomson.

Bothe, A. K., Davidow, J. H., Bramlett, R. E., & Ingham, R. J. (2006) Stuttering treatment research 1970-2005: I. Systematic review incorporating trial quality assessment of behavioral, cognitive, and related approaches. *American Journal of Speech-Language Pathology, 15,* 321-341.

Colcord, R. D., & Adams, M. R. (1979) Voicing duration and vocal SPL changes associated with stuttering reduction during singing. *Journal of Speech and Hearing Research, 22,* 468-479.

Davidow, J. D., Bothe, A. K., Andreatta, R. D., & Ye, J. (2009) Measurement of phonated intervals during four fluency-inducing conditions. *Journal of Speech, Language, and Hearing Research, 52,* 188-205.

Goldiamond, I. (1965) Stuttering and fluency as manipulatable operant response classes. In: L. Krasner & L. P. Ullman (Eds.), *Research in Behavior Modification: New Developments and Implications* (pp. 106-156). New York: Holt, Rinehart and Winston, Inc.

Goldiamond, I. (1967) *Supplementary statement to operant analysis and control of fluent and nonfluent verbal behavior.* Report to Department of Health, Education, and Welfare, Public Health Service Application No. MH-8876-03.

Gow, M. L., & Ingham, R. J. (1992) Modifying electroglottograph-identified intervals of phonation: The effect on stuttering. *Journal of Speech and Hearing Research, 35,* 495-511.

Ingham, R. J. (1980) Modification and maintenance of generalization during stuttering treatment. *Journal of Speech and Hearing Research, 23,* 732-745.

Ingham, R. J. (1982) The effects of self-evaluation training on maintenance and generalization during stuttering treatment. *Journal of Speech and Hearing Disorders, 47,* 271-280.

Ingham, R. J. (1999) Performance-contingent management of stuttering in adolescents and adults. In: R. Curlee (Ed.), *Stuttering and Related Disorders of Fluency* (pp. 200-221). New York: Thieme.

Ingham, R., & Devan, D. (1987) *Phonated and nonphonated interval modifications in the speech of stutterers.* Paper read at the annual meeting of the American Speech-Language-Hearing Association. New Orleans, LA; November.

Ingham, R. J., Ingham, J. C., & Bothe, A. K. (in press) Integrating functional measures with treatment: a tactic for enhancing personally significant change in the treatment of adults and adolescents who stutter. *American Journal of Speech-Language Pathology.*

Ingham, R. J., Ingham, J. C., Finn, P., & Fox, P. T. (2003) Towards a functional neural systems model of developmental stuttering. *Journal of Fluency Disorders, 28,* 297-318.

Ingham, R. J., Kilgo, M., Ingham, J. C., Moglia, R., Belknap, H., & Sanchez, T. (2001) Evaluation of a stuttering treatment based on reduction of short phonation intervals. *Journal of Speech, Language, and Hearing Research, 44,* 1229-1244.

Ingham, R. J, Moglia, R., Kilgo, M., & Felino, A. (2007) *Modifying Phonation Interval (MPI) Stuttering Treatment Program.* Santa Barbara: University of California.

Ingham, R. J., Montgomery, J., & Ulliana, L. (1983) The effect of manipulating phonation duration on stuttering. *Journal of Speech and Hearing Research, 26,* 579–587.

Manning, W. H., & Coufal, K. J. (1976) The frequency of disfluencies during phonatory transitions in stuttered and nonstuttered speech. *Journal of Communication Disorders, 9,* 75–81.

Martin, R. R., Haroldson, S. K., & Triden, K. (1984) Stuttering and speech naturalness. *Journal of Speech and Hearing Disorders, 49,* 53–58.

Onslow, M., & O'Brian, S. (1998) Reliability of clinician's judgments about prolonged-speech targets. *Journal of Speech, Language, and Hearing Research, 41,* 969–975.

Packman, A., Onslow, M., & van Doorn, J. (1994) Prolonged speech modification of stuttering: Perceptual, acoustic, and electroglottographic data. *Journal of Speech and Hearing Research, 37,* 724–737.

Adams, M. R., & Ramig, P. (1980) Vocal characteristics of normal speakers and stutterers during choral reading. *Journal of Speech and Hearing Research, 23,* 457–469.

UCSB. (2010) Stuttering treatment clinic. Retrieved from http://www.speech.ucsb.edu/clinic/.

Wingate, M. E. (1969) Sound and pattern in "artificial" fluency. *Journal of Speech and Hearing Research, 12,* 677–686.

Wingate, M. E. (1970) Effect on stuttering of changes in audition. *Journal of Speech and Hearing Research, 13,* 861–873.

Chapter 2

The Camperdown Program

Sue O'Brian and Brenda Carey

The University of Sydney, Sydney, Australia

Overview

The Camperdown Program (CP), which was named after the Sydney suburb in which it was first trialled, was developed by researchers at the Australian Stuttering Research Centre at The University of Sydney. It is a speech restructuring treatment developed for adults who stutter, but it has also been adapted for adolescents as young as 13 years old. The term speech restructuring refers to the use of 'a new speech pattern to reduce or eliminate stuttering while sounding as natural as possible' (Onslow and Menzies, 2010). The primary aim of the programme is to significantly reduce stuttering during everyday speech situations and to maintain this behaviour change over time. A secondary aim of the treatment is to assist clients to develop self-managed procedures so that they may be able to deal with any stuttering increase after treatment. Although the programme does not directly target speech-related anxiety associated with stuttering, there is flexibility during the treatment to incorporate such procedures if and when they are required.

The programme consists of four stages: (1) teaching the treatment components, (2) instatement of natural-sounding, stutter-free speech within the treatment environment, (3) generalisation of controlled speech into everyday speaking situations and, finally, (4) maintenance of the behaviour change. The programme can be implemented intensively or in weekly clinic visits, in a group or one-on-one with the clinician and face-to-face with a clinician or in telehealth format via webcam or telephone. The manual, clinic forms and video model can be downloaded from the website of the ASRC: http://sydney .edu.au/health_sciences/asrc/health_professionals/asrc_download.shtml

Stage 1: Teaching

The first stage of the CP involves clients learning some basic skills needed to undertake the programme. These include the speech restructuring

---

The Science and Practice of Stuttering Treatment: A Symposium, First Edition. Edited by Suzana Jelčić Jakšić and Mark Onslow.
© 2012 John Wiley & Sons, Ltd. Published 2012 by John Wiley & Sons, Ltd.

technique and the clinical speech measures. The speech measures used in the programme are a 9-point stuttering severity scale, where 1 represents no stuttering and 9 represents extremely severe stuttering, and a 9-point speech naturalness scale, where 1 represents extremely natural speech and 9 represents extremely unnatural speech. Clients learn their new speech technique by imitating a standard video model of the speech delivered in a slow and exaggerated manner.

The severity scale replaces traditional stutter-count measures for three reasons: (1) evidence suggests that there is currently no known standard procedure for identifying and measuring individual stutters reliably, (2) there is an abundance of literature to support severity rating scales being used reliably by both speech pathologists and people who stutter with little or no training and (3) from a purely practical point of view, severity rating scales require no equipment. The speech naturalness scale replaces speech rate measurement throughout the programme. Evidence has confirmed that both speech pathologists and people who stutter can reliably measure speech naturalness with the 9-point scale.

Stage 2: Instatement

During the second or Instatement Stage of the programme, clients aim to establish natural-sounding, stutter-free speech within the treatment environment. This process involves no programmed instruction and no rate control but follows the process established with a laboratory study (Packman et al., 1994). Clients practice their new speech technique during a series of speech cycles. Each cycle consists of three 5-minute phases: (1) a Practice Phase, (2) a Trial Phase and (3) an Evaluation Phase.

During the Practice Phase, clients imitate the video or audio model. They practise speaking in monologue or conversation, aiming for a severity of 1-2 and a speech naturalness of 7-9. They record this practice, and then evaluate their severity and naturalness from the recording. Finally, they receive clinician feedback for the task.

Each Practice Phase is followed by a Trial Phase where clients are encouraged to speak in monologue or conversation using whatever features of the speech pattern they require to control their stuttering. Before speaking, they decide on a naturalness goal they wish to achieve and then aim for a severity rating of 1-2. This trial is audio recorded.

Each Trial Phase is followed by an Evaluation Phase. Here, after listening to the recording of their speech, clients re-evaluate their stuttering severity and their speech naturalness scores. They decide whether their stated goals were met; they consider the acceptability of their speech naturalness and plan a strategy for the next cycle. They may choose to practise the speech pattern some more or to experiment with making their speech sound more natural.

Clients rotate through as many of these cycles as required to meet criteria for the next stage. Clients progress to the Generalisation Stage of the programme when they consistently achieve a stuttering severity score of 1–2 and a speech naturalness score of 1–3 within the treatment environment.

Stage 3: Generalisation

The third or Generalisation Stage of the programme involves the client developing strategies to use stutter-free speech during everyday speaking situations. Clients evaluate their stuttering severity and speech naturalness in individualised and relevant everyday situations. These measures form the basis of problem-solving activities to maximise outcomes. It is during this stage that the addition of simple cognitive behaviour therapy strategies, as outlined by Menzies et al. (2009), may be introduced to address speech-related anxiety.

Stage 4: Maintenance

During the fourth and final stage of the programme, the Maintenance Stage, clients continue to develop problem-solving skills to assist maintenance of their gains. The aim is to reduce reliance on the clinician and to increase client self-reliance to deal with fluctuations in stuttering.

Theoretical basis

The mechanisms underpinning the beneficial effects of speech restructuring treatments are not known. Previous research has suggested that such treatments reduce the variability of syllabic stress. In other words, after practising the speech pattern, syllables tend to be more equally stressed (Packman et al., 1994). So, if it is the case that stuttering is triggered by variable syllabic stress, as has been suggested by one theoretical model (Packman et al., 1996, 2007), then it seems logical that stuttering will decrease when restructured speech is used. However, the CP was not developed from any theoretical position; its development was empirically driven. The procedures used in the programme are supported by evidence from rigorous laboratory studies and from Phase I and II clinical trials research.

Demonstrated value

The empirical evidence underpinning the CP suggests that several of the components, which are typical of traditional speech restructuring treatment programmes, might in fact not be necessary for the successful instatement and generalisation of stutter-free speech. These elements are (1) a standardised, prescriptive, speech pattern (2) programmed instruction to instate natural-sounding, stutter-free speech, (3) formal transfer procedures to aid generalisation and (4) counting of stutters online.

When teaching the speech pattern, no attempt is made to specify its features with traditional terms such as soft contacts for consonants, gentle onsets of vowels and continuous vocalisation. This feature of the programme was based on evidence from two laboratory studies. In the first of these, Packman et al. (1994) showed that adults who stutter could produce natural-sounding, stutter-free speech simply by imitating a slow version of a speech restructuring model. Subsequent acoustic analyses of their speech showed that all participants were using different features of the pattern to control their stuttering. This suggested that adults who stuttered were likely to benefit most from using individualised features of speech restructuring rather than a predetermined, standardised speech pattern. The Packman et al. (1994) report also showed that participants were able to benefit from the speech pattern without any need for programmed instruction.

Further support for the non-specific clinical approach to using a speech pattern came from a study by Onslow and O'Brian (1998). This study shows that speech pathologists have difficulty agreeing not only about whether clients are using soft contacts and gentle onsets correctly but even whether they are using them at all. This lack of agreement of course would make consistent teaching using such terms virtually impossible and suggested that correct use of such behaviours by clients, therefore, may not be essential to the outcomes of the programme. Another feature of the CP is that there are no formal hierarchical transfer tasks because omission of these was shown to be viable with a clinical trial by Harrison et al. (1998). The absence of any formal, online counting of stuttering events during the CP is based on a large body of research indicating problems with such a procedure (e.g. Bothe, 2008; Brundage et al., 2006; Ingham and Cordes, 1992; Kully and Boberg, 1988).

Evidence for the efficacy of the CP comes from outcomes from over 100 participants in seven published clinical trials, including Phase I and II studies, and a randomised controlled trial, with medium-term follow-up.

The first study was a Phase I trial with three adults (O'Brian et al., 2001). A Phase I trial is a preliminary investigation designed to test the viability and the safety of a programme and to confirm the treatment protocol. All three adults completed the programme and attained maintenance criteria in a mean of 18 clinic hours. Ten to thirteen months after beginning treatment, all had attained and maintained less than 1% stuttered syllables in beyond-clinic speaking situations. The group mean percent stuttering reduction was 90.4%. These results confirmed a potential treatment effect and justified proceeding to a Phase II trial.

The second study was a non-randomised Phase II trial designed to assess the number of treatment responders (O'Brian et al., 2003). This trial recruited 30 participants. The 21 who attained maintenance criteria did so in a mean of 20 clinic hours. The primary outcome measure for this study was percentage of syllables stuttered during beyond-clinic speaking situations up to 12 months post-treatment. Results demonstrated a 95% group mean stuttering reduction from pre-treatment to 12 months post-treatment, although there was significant individual variation (Figure 2.1). Group mean speech

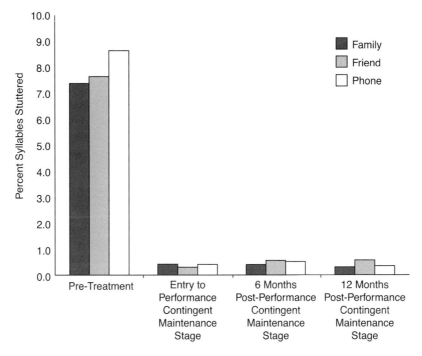

Figure 2.1 Stuttering frequency in percent syllables stuttered during four assessments beyond the clinic. Adapted by permission of the American Speech-Language-Hearing Association.

naturalness scores for these adults were within one scale score of matched controls. Self-report and social validity measures mostly confirmed the outcomes.

Further support for the treatment comes from outcomes of Phase I and Phase II trials of the treatment adapted for telehealth delivery (Carey et al., 2010; O'Brian et al., 2008). Participants in those trials did not attend the clinic. Instead, the treatment was conducted remotely with contact occurring only by telephone and e-mail. We will present details of these studies in Chapter 10. However, these two trials, consisting of 53 participants, produced group mean reductions in stuttering of 66% and around 82%, respectively, with the number of clinician hours decreasing still further to an average of between 10–12.

Although designed to be used with the adult population, the programme has also been trialled with adolescents. Hearne et al. (2008) conducted a Phase I trial with three adolescents aged 13, 14 and 16 years. In this trial, no significant adaptations were made to accommodate the younger population. The oldest of the three children responded very well, reducing his stuttering to below 1% and maintaining this result for at least 12 months. However, the younger two children did not perform as well. Subsequent modifications have recently been made to the programme to make it more suitable for this age group. A recent Phase I trial of a Skype Internet version (Carey et al., in press) shows significantly improved outcomes for adolescents, with a group mean percent stuttering reduction of 92% at 6 months post-treatment.

Finally, a clinical trial of the treatment with adults but delivered by students under supervision (Cocomazzo et al., in press) has confirmed that similar results can be achieved under those conditions. The 12 participants in this trial achieved a mean 62% reduction in stuttering 12 months after treatment.

In summary, there is strong evidence from Phase I and Phase II clinical trials with adults and adolescents that the CP can produce significant reductions in stuttering regardless of the delivery format. That evidence is robust because outcomes have been collected from both objective and self-report measures, supported by speech naturalness data, in everyday speaking situations, independent of the treatment environment and for up to 12 months after treatment. Outcomes have been shown to be socially valid during this research.

Advantages and disadvantages

Advantages

The CP has a number of advantages over traditional speech restructuring programmes. The most obvious is the reduced clinician time required to achieve comparable outcomes. This programme requires a mean of around 10-20 clinic hours depending on the treatment delivery model. This is a substantial saving compared to the 50 or even 100 plus hours required for more traditional intensive group programmes that may even include a residential component.

The CP allows for flexibility of treatment delivery. For example, it can be administered entirely at a distance, using phone or webcam technology allowing equity of access particularly for remotely located people. It can also be offered in group or individual format, hence catering for different client preferences and infrastructure needs.

The programme has been manualised for implementation by generalist clinicians. It requires no specialist skills, no equipment and it can be delivered by whatever method is suited to a clinician's caseload. Taking the service away from specialist centres again allows for greater access to treatment for the general population.

Disadvantages

The disadvantages of the programme are those that are inherent to all speech restructuring programmes. The learning of a new speech pattern requires effort and focus to maintain over long periods. Relapse is common and speech that sounds and feels unnatural to some extent seems inevitable. The limitations to the CP evidence also need to be acknowledged. There has been no replication of these findings independently of our research group. Further, there has been no investigation of the treatment against a 'no treatment' control group. As such, it is likely that the effect sizes have been overestimated (Kunz and Oxman, 1998). There have been no long-term follow-up studies past 12 months and given the well-acknowledged relapse rates with adult stuttering treatments, this is also a caveat to the findings.

Conclusions and future direction

In conclusion, the CP is a speech restructuring treatment for which there is reasonable empirical evidence for both its treatment processes and its efficacy. So what does the future hold for the programme? We are just completing a Phase I trial of a completely clinician-free, Internet-based version that clients complete in their own time, and in their own environments (Erickson et al., 2012). This version retains all the concepts of the original programme but clients work through the programme at their own pace. This will obviously not be the solution for all clients; however, preliminary data have shown that it is a viable model for some. Hopefully in the future, we will be able to report on a model that makes treatment accessible to anyone, wherever and whenever they need it. How satisfying that would be for both the stuttering population and for speech pathologists!

Discussion

Ann Packman
Our group was interested that you reported variable outcomes for clients in the trials.

Sue O'Brian
I don't know whether many of you noticed that the outcomes for the earlier trials were better than the outcomes for the later trials. What happened from the first trials to the later trials is that we changed the way we measured outcomes. For the earlier trials, although outcomes were measured beyond the clinic, in three different situations – friend, telephone and family – all of those beyond-clinic outcome measures were client initiated and that obviously is a bit of a problem. If participants are able to initiate their own assessment situations, then they can potentially manipulate outcomes. In the later trials, they were still beyond-clinic measures, but we did not allow the participants to initiate the assessments – we had 'surprise' phone calls to participants. Surprise is a bit of a loose term. Obviously, they are not surprise calls in the sense that participants did not know they were coming, but they were surprise calls in the sense that they did not know when they would come. We always have to establish a convenient window of time for when the participants can take the calls so there is some known element. These surprise calls are from two strangers, who are researchers at the Australian Stuttering Research Centre. The procedure has the advantage that participants cannot rehearse

before an assessment phone call and they cannot choose who the call will be from. And most importantly, they cannot remake a recording if they are not happy with the first recording. Now I don't know if that has ever happened, but we sometimes wondered with the way we used to collect outcome recordings. So the way that we are now collecting objective stuttering-count assessments is a much more valid way of doing it. So for that reason I think probably the outcomes the later trials provide are a more valid effect size estimate than the earlier trials.

Ann Packman

I wonder if you could give some idea of predictors of those outcomes? How useful were severity or previous treatment, or other factors, as predictors?

Sue O'Brian

There have been no studies to date that have specifically explored predictors of outcome. However, for a number of the trials we have explored correlates of outcome. None of our studies so far have recruited enough subjects to allow statistically useful predictors of outcome, but we have at least looked at correlates. Nothing has come up. Severity, previous treatment and family history have not been correlates of outcome for our trials. But of course you need to take that as a preliminary finding only. Sophisticated regression modelling, when we have sufficient numbers, may provide a different result.

Sheena Reilly

Sue, I think the first comment our group made was what a great example it was of building evidence about a programme and approach, so congratulations from the group. During the Instatement Stage, how do you get from the imitation task during the Practice Phase to shaping speech naturalness during the Trial Phase? How do you decide which speech components you're going to work on to make speech natural?

Sue O'Brian

The way it's taught in the first place is just by exposure to the video model during the Practice Phase. What we do clinically is play the video or the audio for clients, get them to listen to it a few times and try to imitate it. Clinicians often ask how you give feedback about the speech pattern without using traditional terms to instruct clients such as 'soft contacts', 'gentle onsets', 'continuous vocalisation', and so on. It is easy to break the video model into small bits and compare that small bit with the attempted client production. Often, we will tape record the client and compare the two small bits of the model, asking, 'How do you think it sounds? Can you make yourself sound more like that?' What we find is that clients don't have any problem with that, as long as the model is broken down into smaller bits and they copy it bit by bit. We don't insist clinically that clients imitate the model exactly (unless they want to) because that would fly in the face of the underlying assumptions of the programme.

Joseph Attanasio

Is there a resistance to go into an unnatural speech pattern, and if so how do you overcome that?

Sue O'Brian

No, because what we want the clients to do during the Practice Phase is to develop their own individual pattern that completely controls their stuttering. So if in the Practice Phase of the programme they develop a technique or a pattern that seems to be completely controlling their stuttering, we will ask them, 'Do you feel like you could stutter? At all?' No. 'Okay, then that's the technique' – the pattern, whatever you want to call it – 'that's the one that's going to help you.' Once clients get to that level during the Practice Phase, then that's the first stage of the programme, where you have them at a very unnatural level using a speech restructuring technique where they feel they are completely in control of their stuttering, where there is no room for any stuttering whatsoever. If they are using a speech restructuring technique well they will not stutter at all. When we get that far then we go into the Trial Phase where the cycles happen and they start to shape more natural-sounding speech while retaining control of stuttering.

Sheena Reilly

Can you just clarify the procedures?

Sue O'Brian

Clients cycle through the three phases: Practice, Trial and Evaluation. During the Practice Phase, they are just imitating the video with speech naturalness 7-9, which is extremely unnatural. During Trial Phase they move from imitation of the video to monologue and conversation with the clinician, and they are told to use any features of the pattern that they think they need to control stuttering while attempting to make their speech sound more natural. There is no programmed instruction. In other words, we don't use the traditional approach of starting at, say, 40 syllables a minute and moving to 70 syllables a minute to 100 syllables a minute, and so on, or starting at naturalness 9, and moving systematically from naturalness 8, to 7, to 6, and so on. Instead, we allow clients to just use the features as they please. They set their own speech naturalness targets. They know their goal in a Trial Phase is a severity of 1-2, so its got to be virtually no stuttering or no stuttering at all, and they set a naturalness target that they think they can achieve to meet that goal. So every client does it differently. You will get those clients who want to play it safe and they'll stay at a very unnatural level for quite a long time. Such 'play it safe' clients have the same speech naturalness during the Trial Phase as they did in the Practice Phase, because they want to reinforce their speech technique. You'll get others who are more adventurous and say: 'Okay, if I'm allowed to set my naturalness, I want to sound really natural, so I'm going for a naturalness 3.' Then what happens in such cases, nine out of ten times, is that they will stutter during the Trial Phase and during the subsequent Evaluation Phase, when they evaluate their speech from the recording, they will hear how little of the speech restructuring technique they are using and they will reset their strategies, aiming for less natural speech, with more technique, during the next Trial Phase so that they do not stutter. Then you get others who pace themselves evenly throughout the cycles and move progressively from higher to lower naturalness scores during the Trial Phases. And finally you get other kinds of clients who go up and down with their speech naturalness during the Trial Phases, and rely a lot on problem solving, saying: 'Okay, this is what I did this time, my severity was this, my naturalness was that, I wasn't happy with that; this time I'm going to set a goal and I'm going to do that.'

Joseph Attanasio

Now to a different issue. You mention in your presentation and in your publications that the CP is not based on any theoretical model and the group was wondering might it be incorrect to say that? Surely motor control theory underlies CP because after all you are slowing down speech, you are changing motoric aspects of speech, and might not that be at the core of this and so might it be theoretically driven?

Sue O'Brian

First of all, there is evidence for how speech restructuring might work. There's evidence to show that, for example, the variability of vowel duration decreases with speech restructuring patterns. And if you consider theories such as those I mention, they would explain why the speech restructuring process works. The thing I am keen to promote is that it was not a theory that drove the development of the programme; empirical studies drove the development of the programme. We did so looking at the laboratory evidence I mentioned, in particular the Packman et al. (1994) study.

Ann Packman

Sue, our group was interested that you mentioned using cognitive behaviour therapy procedures during the Problem Solving Stage. Could you elaborate on what they are and do you think that an unskilled or an untrained therapist could do them?

Sue O'Brian

The first thing I need to say is that the primary CP goal is to reduce or eliminate stuttering. But of course that does not mean that speech-related anxiety should be overlooked. That would just be silly, considering the evidence about the number of adults who stutter and seek speech treatment that have speech-related anxiety. I imagine most speech pathologists would assess speech-related anxiety when they do an assessment.

We use a couple of different tools for assessing anxiety, one being the UTBAS scale that is an acronym for Unhelpful Thoughts and Beliefs about Stuttering (Iverach et al., 2011; St Clare et al., 2008). The UTBAS scale is a 60-item checklist, which was developed by psychologists working with adults who stutter. It was taken from a file audit of clinical cases and established the unhelpful thoughts and beliefs that adults who stutter typically present in a treatment environment. I think it is a useful tool, not for diagnosing anxiety but for finding out what sort of anxiety, the levels of anxiety and what sort of situations clients fear. It contains a series of statements and asks clients to indicate the extent to which each applies to them: for example, 'I feel stupid when I stutter' and 'people will laugh at me when I stutter'. Those unhelpful cognitions are used during the Problem Solving Stage of the CP. The other tool that we often use is the fear of negative evaluation scale (Watson and Friend, 1969). So those tools give you a lot of information to use during the treatment process. I tend to find that anxiety becomes a problem most often during the problem-solving components of the programme – not always, but mostly, as that is when clients want to generalise their stutter-free speech into real world speaking situations.

A publication by Menzies et al. (2009) provides basic cognitive behaviour therapy strategies for use by those who feel professionally qualified to do so. But the caveat here is that cognitive behaviour therapy is the domain of clinical psychologists, not speech pathologists. That being said, I do think many adults who stutter who seek stuttering control would benefit from cognitive behaviour therapy. How speech pathologists might present those services is a topic to which I don't think time will allow me to digress.

Sheena Reilly

Our group discussed the advantages of the CP flexibility for individual clients. Obviously you are an experienced clinician and your team developed the programme. But how suitable is it for generalist clinicians, particularly in the telehealth and Internet-based versions you mentioned.

Sue O'Brian

The short answer is that the manual has been written with generalist clinicians in mind, so it's written as a simplistic step-by-step programme. The skills required are not those of a specialist clinician. First, there is no counting of stuttering moments. The CP just uses a severity rating scale. And second, because the video model is provided, it is possible for a clinician to do the treatment without having to constantly provide perfect demonstrations of the target speech pattern; the video model does that. I also think that telehealth is no problem, but we will get to that later (see Chapter 10).

Sheena Reilly

I think the question was more about if you didn't have access to a clinician and you were simply doing a standalone Internet-based version.

Sue O'Brian

One of the reasons I am guessing – or hoping – that clinical trials will show a standalone Internet version to be viable is that there is a lot of drill with the programme. Our Phase I trial (Erickson et al., 2012) show that some clients can use the Internet version satisfactorily.

Joe Attanasio

Our group had a concern about your comment that the CP can be done without specialised training. And there was also a concern about how outcomes were judged. We queried the reliability and freedom from bias in the outcome assessment process and that is an issue that you might want to clarify at some point.

Sue O'Brian

Hopefully, at some time we will have an empirical response to your first concern. Regarding the second concern, all of us who conduct stuttering treatment research are tarred by that brush.

References

Bothe, A. K. (2008) Identification of children's stuttered and nonstuttered speech by highly experienced judges: Binary judgements and comparisons with disfluency-types definitions. *Journal of Speech, Language, and Hearing Research, 51,* 867–878.

Brundage, S. B., Bothe, A. K., Lengeling, A. N., & Evans, J. J. (2006) Comparing judgments of stuttering made by students, clinicians, and highly experienced judges. *Journal of Fluency Disorders, 31,* 271–283.

Carey, B., O'Brian, S., Onslow, M., Block, S., Jones, M., & Packman, A. (2010) Randomized controlled non-inferiority trial of a telehealth treatment for chronic stuttering: the Camperdown Program. *International Journal of Language and Communication Disorders, 45,* 108–120.

Carey, B., O'Brian, S., Onslow, M., Packman, A., & Menzies, R. (in press) Webcam delivery of the Camperdown Program for adolescents who stutter: a Phase I trial. *Language Speech and Hearing Services in Schools.*

Cocomazzo, N., Block, S., Carey, B., O'Brian, S., & Onslow, M. (in press) Camperdown Program for adults who stutter: a student training clinic Phase I trial. *International Journal of Language and Communication Disorders.*

Erickson, S., Block, S., Menzies, R., Onslow, M., O'Brian, S., & Packman, A. (2012) Standalone Internet speech restructuring treatment for adults who stutter: a Phase I trial. Manuscript in preparation.

Harrison, E., Onslow, M., Andrews, C., Packman, A., & Webber, M. (1998) Control of stuttering with prolonged speech: Development of a one-day instatement program. In: A. K. Cordes & R. J. E. Ingham (Eds.), *Treatment Efficacy in Stuttering.* San Diego, CA: Singular Publishing.

Hearne, A., Packman, A., Onslow, M., & O'Brian, S. (2008) Developing treatment for adolescents who stutter: a Phase I trial of the Camperdown Program. *Language, Speech, and Hearing Services in School, 39,* 487–497.

Ingham, R. J., & Cordes, A. K. (1992) Interclinic differences in stuttering-event counts. *Journal of Fluency Disorders, 17,* 171–176.

Iverach, L., Menzies, R., Jones, M., O'Brian, S., Packman, A., & Onslow, M. (2011) Further development and validation of the Unhelpful Thoughts and Beliefs About Stuttering (UTBAS) scales: relationship to anxiety and social phobia among adults who stutter. *International Journal of Language and Communication Disorders, 46,* 286–299.

Kully, D., & Boberg, E. (1988) An investigation of interclinic agreement in the identification of fluent and stuttered syllables. *Journal of Fluency Disorders, 13,* 309–318.

Kunz, R., & Oxman, A. (1998) The unpredictability paradox: review of empirical comparisons of randomised and non-randomised clinical trials. *British Medical Journal, 317,* 1185–1190.

Menzies, R. G., Onslow, M., Packman, A., & O'Brian, S. (2009) Cognitive behavior therapy for adults who stutter: a tutorial for speech-language pathologists. *Journal of Fluency Disorders, 34,* 187–200.

O'Brian, S., Cream, A., Onslow, M., & Packman, A. (2001) A replicable, non-programmed, instrument-free method for the control of stuttering with prolonged speech. Papers from the 2nd Asia Pacific Conference on Speech, Language and Hearing, Part IV. *Asia Pacific Journal of Speech, Language and Hearing, 6*(2), 91–96.

O'Brian, S., Onslow, M., Cream, A., & Packman, A. (2003) The Camperdown Program: outcomes of a new prolonged-speech treatment model. *Journal of Speech, Language, and Hearing Research, 46,* 933–946.

O'Brian, S., Packman, A., & Onslow, M. (2008) Telehealth delivery of the Camperdown Program for adults who stutter: a Phase I Trial. *Journal of Speech, Language, and Hearing Research, 51,* 184–195.

Onslow, M., & Menzies, R. (2010) Speech restructuring. Accepted entry in www.commonlanguagepsychotherapy.org

Onslow, M., & O'Brian, S. (1998) Reliability of clinicians' judgments about prolonged-speech targets. *Journal of Speech, Language, and Hearing Research, 41,* 969–975.

Packman, A., Code, C., & Onslow, M. (2007) On the cause of stuttering: Integrating theory with brain and behavioral research. *Journal of Neurolinguistics, 20,* 353–362.

Packman, A., Onslow, M., Richard, F., & van Doorn, J. (1996) Syllabic stress and variability: a model of stuttering. *Clinical Linguistics and Phonetics, 10,* 235–263.

Packman, A., Onslow, M., & van Doorn, J. (1994) Prolonged speech and modification of stuttering: perceptual, acoustic, and electroglottographic data. *Journal of Speech and Hearing Research, 37,* 724–737.

St Clare, T., Menzies, R., Onslow, M., Packman, A., Thompson, R., & Block, S. (2008) Unhelpful thoughts and beliefs linked to social anxiety in stuttering: development of a measure. *International Journal of Language and Communication Disorders, 44,* 338–351.

Watson, D., & Friend, R. (1969) Measurement of social-evaluative anxiety. *Journal of Consulting and Clinical Psychology, 33,* 448–457.

Chapter 3

Assessment and Treatment of Stuttering Using Altered Auditory Feedback

Tim Saltuklaroglu
University of Tennessee, Knoxville, TX, USA

Overview

The most common forms of altered auditory feedback (AAF) are (1) delayed auditory feedback (DAF), in which users hear their own speech with a slight delay and (2) frequency altered feedback (FAF), in which users hear their own voices with an upwards or downwards shift in pitch. The effects of DAF on speech have been investigated since the 1950s when it was observed that they could produce dysfluency in normal speakers (Lee, 1951) and induce fluency in people who stutter (PWS) (Chase et al., 1961). Therapies for stuttering began to incorporate DAF using longer delays, greater than 200 ms, finding that it induced fluency along with a slowed speech rate (Goldiamond, 1965). When it was discovered that a slowed rate by itself was *sufficient* for inducing fluency, DAF began to be discounted as a therapy option in favour of behavioural rate reduction protocols (Ingham, 1993). Howell et al. (1987) first reported the positive effects of FAF on stuttering. Later, Kalinowski and colleagues conducted a series of studies demonstrating that both DAF and FAF could reduce stuttering at normal and fast speech rates, effectively proving that slowed speech was *not necessary* for reducing stuttering and that the auditory effects of AAF may also be *sufficient* to induce fluent speech in many who stutter (Hargrave et al., 1994; Kalinowski and Stuart, 1996; Stuart et al., 2002).

Technological and theoretical advancements have spurred the resurgence of AAF. Large, bulky AAF devices have given way to more portable and inconspicuous ones, including ear-level devices (e.g. SpeechEasy) and economical computer software applications (e.g. Apple iPhone).

The Science and Practice of Stuttering Treatment: A Symposium, First Edition. Edited by Suzana Jelčić Jakšić and Mark Onslow.
© 2012 John Wiley & Sons, Ltd. Published 2012 by John Wiley & Sons, Ltd.

Theoretical basis

There is considerable evidence from the neuroscience literature indicating strong associations between sensory and motor processes related to speech processing (e.g. Tremblay and Small, 2011). Further, stuttering may be the result of deficits in internal modeling (Max et al., 2004), which may contribute to the observed aberrant activity in cortical centres associated with both speech production and audition (Fox et al., 1996). Hence, when considering the use of AAF from both theoretical and clinical perspectives, it may be appropriate to adopt an integrative approach, which considers the influence that changes in audition can have on production, and vice versa. Simply put, fluency enhancements that appear to be peripherally derived via manipulations in either auditory feedback or motor speech production most likely synergistically alter neurophysiological functioning centrally in regions related both to audition and speech production (Kalinowski and Saltuklaroglu, 2003).

Though much remains to be learned about stuttering, its impact on central speech perception and production mechanisms, and how these mechanisms might be altered to promote fluency, one condition stands out for invariably producing fluent speech in PWS. This condition is choral speech (CS), in which two people speak the same material in unison. Under this condition, stuttering is drastically reduced or eliminated by 90–100%. This robust effect is produced immediately and requires no training or volitional adjustments to speech production (Kalinowski and Saltuklaroglu, 2003). Therefore, it is often considered the highest standard of fluency achievement in PWS. Simply put, it demonstrates that under certain conditions, PWS are capable of producing effortless and natural-sounding fluent speech.

Hence, it is suggested that the power of AAF for reducing stuttering resides in its capacity to emulate CS. This comparison is made because listening to an electronically generated rendition of one's own voice while speaking with AAF is akin to speaking in unison with another speaker (Hargrave et al., 1994). However, a quintessential difference between the two fluency enhancers is the source of the 'second' speaker. Using AAF requires a speaker to produce speech in order for it to be 'fed back' and create the second speaker. In other words, generation of the second speaker is dependent on the presence of a primary speech signal, the speech of the PWS. Logically, this implies that AAF cannot effectively reduce stuttering until speech has been initiated and the PWS is able to hear the electronic speech signal. In contrast, in CS the two speech sources are created independently of each other, meaning that so long as the second speaker is present, the PWS can fluently 'join in'.

Fluent speech initiation is often difficult for those who stutter. Therefore, considering the obligatory role of initiating speech to generate an AAF signal, it stands to reason that initiation difficulties may not be amenable to correction with AAF alone. A recent study examined the relative frequencies of stuttering in the initial syllable and subsequent syllables of 10-second

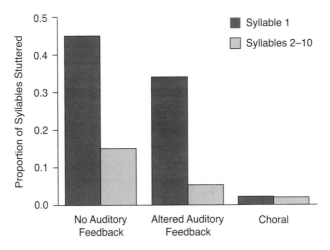

Figure 3.1 Proportions of stuttered syllables on the first syllable and nine subsequent syllables of 10-second utterances in non-altered feedback, altered auditory feedback and choral speech conditions (Saltuklaroglu et al., 2009).

productions under non-altered feedback (NAF), AAF and choral speaking conditions (Saltuklaroglu et al., 2009). Figure 3.1 shows the results. Across conditions AAF reduced stuttering by 68% compared to NAF. However, substantial initiation difficulties, with large proportions of stuttering on the initial syllable, were pervasive across NAF and AAF conditions, demonstrating that fluency enhancement via AAF did not occur until after the initial syllable was spoken. In contrast, CS (during which participants simply 'joined in' speaking with an existing second speaker) produced a 98% reduction in stuttering compared to NAF, with its effects undifferentiated by syllable locus.

These findings highlight the need for many clients who stutter to use motor strategies to synergistically supplement or complement AAF. Initiation strategies such as vowel or voiced continuant elongation of the initial syllable, gentle onsets or even the production of a vocalic starting gesture appear to be good strategies when used in conjunction with AAF. Because breaks in the feedback after speech initiation might also be detrimental to the fluency-enhancing capacities of AAF, those with long, silent blockages might also require the use of motor strategies to help maintain continuous feedback. Kalinowski and Saltuklaroglu (2006) have recommended intermittent vowel prolongation to help maintain the feedback derived via AAF. However, these are but two examples of how motor strategies might be used synergistically with AAF to better enhance fluency. Currently there is no standard prescription for how these and similar strategies might be implemented concurrently with AAF to produce the best combination of fluency, natural-sounding speech and ease of use. However, the simple goal of this synergistic approach is the best possible emulation of CS. Of course, clinical testing of any such protocols are warranted, though it seems logical to suspect that ultimately, optimal combinations of AAF and motor strategies will vary based on their individual needs and expectations.

Demonstrated value

Reductions in stuttering frequency

A large body of data exists demonstrating that stuttering can be immediately and effectively reduced by 50–85% while reading under the effects of AAF. Though a number of studies have also found substantial decreases in stuttering in monologue and conversational tasks (e.g. Antipova et al., 2008; Stuart et al., 2006), the effects are generally not as robust as when reading and seem to be more variable across individuals (Lincoln et al., 2010). Lincoln et al. (2006) reviewed many of the studies examining changes in stuttering frequency under AAF, which may be considered Phase I clinical evidence according to the criteria outlined by Robey (2004). However, there is little evidence of efficacy data collected in more naturalistic extra-clinical settings. Pollard et al. (2009) recently attempted to address this need by measuring the effects of the SpeechEasy device on stuttering frequency in an ABA design using extra-clinical reading, monologue and a question-asking task. Though the authors reported no treatment effect after 4 months of use, their findings have been questioned based on their definition of stuttering, variable participant compliance to the protocol, under-sampling in the question task and the fact that their self-report data were considerably more positive (Saltuklaroglu et al., 2010). As such, there still appears to be a paucity of compelling data directly measuring changes in the stuttering frequencies under AAF in extra-clinical settings and there is a continuing need for research in this domain.

Reduced duration of stuttered events

AAF has also been found to reduce the duration of residual stuttering (Stuart et al., 2008), indicating an overall decrease in severity of remaining stuttered events. In other words, much like the presence of stuttering can contaminate the perceptually fluent utterances of those who stutter (Armson and Kalinowski, 1994), general increases in surrounding fluency can also impact perceptually stuttered speech, perhaps calling into question the manner in which we routinely measure stuttering.

Speech naturalness improvements

Improved speech naturalness is observed when those who stutter use AAF, presumably because of the increased fluency. In addition, it has also been found to be better when fluency is derived using AAF than when derived via fluency shaping, suggesting that the continuous use of motor strategies may impart an unnatural quality on speech (Stuart and Kalinowski, 2004). However, when motor strategies are only used intermittently with AAF, speech naturalness remains improved compared to NAF conditions, suggesting that intermittent use of motor strategies can be used without a detrimental effect on speech naturalness (Stuart et al., 2006).

Positive self-report data

Though there are few studies objectively measuring the effects of AAF in extra-clinical environments, self-report data, which captures the more experiential nature of stuttering and treatment efficacy, continues to suggest that AAF is effective in everyday communication. After using AAF presented with the SpeechEasy device for an average of 6.8 hours per day for 6 months, 105 users reported improvements in overall fluency in conversation and while using the telephone. Additionally they reported improved speech naturalness, decreased avoidances and strong overall satisfaction levels (Kalinowski et al., 2004).

Early work has begun (Cook and Smith, 2006; Molt, 2006; Runyan et al., 2006) investigating if use of the SpeechEasy promotes increased confidence and decreased anxiety and avoidance. If that proves to be the case, these added benefits might not be directly reflected in frequency counts of stuttered syllables. However, it is possible to speculate that they may have more of a positive global impact on speech naturalness, duration of stuttered events and the debilitative cognitive and emotional aspects of stuttering.

Advantages and disadvantages

Advantages

The primary and most attractive feature of AAF is the immediacy of its potent fluency-enhancing effects. Compared to other treatment methods, relatively stable, fluent and natural-sounding speech can be achieved in a shorter period, with a reduced role for extended therapy.

With the improved access to AAF systems, speech-language pathologists conducting stuttering assessments can immediately test the potential AAF has for reducing stuttering in almost any client. They can quickly examine how its effects work in isolation and often how best to synergistically combine AAF use with motor techniques for optimal fluency enhancement in a variety of speaking environments, including extra-clinical settings. Simultaneously, they can address clients' immediate reactions to AAF, their perceptions of the resultant speech and help determine if AAF might be a suitable therapeutic option.

The benefits of AAF appear to extend beyond the realm of fluency, as evident by positive self-reports describing declining negative impact of the covert experiential aspects of stuttering such as avoidance and anxiety.

As suggested previously, AAF may best be used when combined with motor speech strategies. However, depending on individual needs, there are numerous possibilities for combining AAF, as either a primary or secondary therapeutic modality, with combinations of behavioural and cognitive therapies.

Disadvantages

Whereas the powerful effects of CS appear pervasive, it is clear that AAF does not reduce stuttering to the same robust extent in everyone who stutters. It is still unclear why this is the case and could be related to multiple factors including severity, individual patterns of stuttering, ability to initiate and maintain speech, age, ability to respond to an AAF signal, therapy history and possibly even different sub-types of stuttering (Antipova et al., 2008). Clearly more investigation is warranted to help evaluate the influence of these factors on fluency enhancement via AAF.

Because AAF offers the advantage of producing more immediate and natural-sounding speech than other methods, intervention periods may be shorter with a smaller role for the speech-language pathologist. As such, therapy with AAF often targets fluency alone. Consequently, little attention may be paid to the cognitive and emotional aspects of stuttering. Though self-report evidence suggest that improvements in these areas may be associated with AAF use, in general AAF focuses on decreasing overt stuttering behaviours rather than the covert experiential aspects, which if left unattended, might remain and continue to hinder communication. As such, it is recommended that speech-language pathologists using AAF educate clients regarding the possible need for additional therapy to cope with the covert emotional components of stuttering.

Questions arise whether long-term exposure to AAF may result in habituation to the signal, such that its fluency enhancement diminishes over time. Though Stuart et al. (2006) found that the positive effects of AAF did not diminish after 4 and 12 months post-treatment, their protocol included the use of motor strategies in conjunction with AAF. Still, as relapse after therapy is a common concern in treatments for stuttering, the possibility of habituation should be considered, especially if used without motor supplementation. However, it may be difficult to differentiate habituation effects from diminished attention to the signal and as such, attentional factors should be considered prior to making judgments about habitation. If diminishing effects are observed, they might be explained by current technologies failing to produce a continuously potent rendition of CS, rather than PWS not using a prescribed technique to enhance the effects. Future renditions of AAF are expected to provide more powerful and dynamic emulations of CS that would likely be more resistant to potential habituation effects. In current forms, frequent manipulations of DAF and FAF parameters, along with reminders to simultaneously implement motor strategies and attend to the signal, might be helpful for maintaining fluency gains over time.

Though many anecdotal reports exist of 'carry-over' fluency, such as continued improvements in fluency after AAF is removed, there is still little documented evidence that this might occur (Van Borsel et al., 2003). Thus, in order to maintain the effects of AAF, it appears that continued use of an external device to provide the signal is necessary.

Conclusions and future directions

The documented positive effects of AAF provide a strong impetus for continuing the evaluation of all its benefits in the remediation of stuttering. Measures should address changes across the entire stuttering syndrome, including naturalness, stuttering durations, and covert aspects of stuttering, along with stuttering frequencies. AAF should optimally be used in conjunction with motor strategies to complement and enhance the AAF signal, with the goal to emulate CS. Applied in this manner, the use of AAF can help provide effective and efficient fluency enhancement and serve as a strong catalyst for managing stuttering. Because of previous limitations in its method of delivery, its application in extra-clinical settings is relatively new and a great deal remains to be learned about the driving force behind the positive effects and how it can best be harnessed to best benefit clients who stutter across a multitude of speaking environments. Considering that technological advancements are forthcoming, it seems logical to conclude that the use of AAF in the treatment of stuttering is in its infancy and we should be optimistic about the potential treatment options it will provide in the future.

Continued research would be expected to provide a better understanding of interactions between speech and audition, their role in the nature and remediation of stuttering and factors contributing to the success or failure of AAF protocols in the management of stuttering.

Perhaps the most exciting prospect for AAF treatments is that improving technologies will surely lead to improvement in the electronic signal. In addition to improved second signals with fewer ambient noise problems, future versions of AAF may provide options for more dynamic signals and possibility of acoustic 'gestural' supplementation to silent periods to aid in speech initiation or when the second signal is halted by long silent blockages.

Discussion

Joseph Attanasio

Your presentation raised the question of how to combine such devices with more traditional treatment approaches. Can you expand on that?

Tim Saltuklaroglu

The methods I use (combinations of AAF and prolonged speech) have not been tested scientifically. I am using them intuitively and this is what I find works for me. The first thing I do is find out if AAF has the potential to help, so I will introduce a client to AAF in a gradual way by fitting the device, having them say some vowels, counting days of the week and months of the year gradually until they build up to reading passages. I get a feel for how much it is helping during reading. Based on the improvement I see during reading with the types of stuttering people are exhibiting, I introduce some intermittent prolongation. There are different ways I do that. Sometimes it is to put a prolonged vowel every third or fourth word. If that seems to help I'll try to find an even balance. The idea is to introduce some prolongation to improve and maintain fluency and speech naturalness. If there are any particular hard sounds for clients I might instruct them to stretch the vowel just before that hard sound. Another strategy – and I like to us this myself[1] – is to have clients stretch a few function words, such as 'in', 'and' and 'on'. That is because, typically, with increasing age stuttering occurs less on function words compared to content words. Function words are short with strong vowels so I can do that without compromising naturalness too much. So that's another intermittent prolongation strategy that I try for my clients and myself. Once clients are comfortable at a reading level using some type of vowel prolongation with comfortable fluency and natural-sounding speech, I will take them to the next level and try conversational tasks. Eventually I have them use the AAF device outside in the real world where they can see it works for them in a more natural setting and against some background noise. The process will vary with every client. I would not want to prescribe a 'recipe' for it. I think the important thing when using AAF is to understand how the signal works and how you can combine that clinically with prolongation in a flexible manner.

Sheena Reilly

Is there any evidence about the use of different types of AAF for conversational speech. We ask because the data that you presented to us is very much about reading tasks and it showed fine results there. But what sort of data exists for conversational speech? Also, our group were interested in whether people might be experiencing merely a placebo effect from using such devices?

Tim Saltuklaroglu

There has been less done with conversational speech than reading. However, recently The Australian Stuttering Research Centre group has reported on conversational speech (Lincoln et al., 2010) and there have been some other reports. The general finding is that fluency enhancement is not as strong as when reading and it varies from person to person. Some clients do quite well with conversation and others do not. I believe that is because of the difference in the tasks. During conversational speech there is the added demands of thinking, formulating and starting and stopping.[2] I have seen clients who can do wonderfully with AAF during a reading task because all they do is focus on

---

[1]Dr Saltuklaroglu is a person who stutters.
[2]Dr Saltuklaroglu is describing how conversational speech in effect requires dual tasking.

speech. But then during conversation these added demands make it a different task altogether. I think more research is needed to determine how to improve the effects of these devices in conversation.

Related to this issue is what the observers were asking me while your groups where meeting; see Preface for an explanation of who the observers were. How do we know it's the acoustic signal or a speech signal? We've compared the effects of speech and non-speech signals (Dayalu et al., 2011; Kalinowski et al., 2000). With tones or even fricative speech sounds you don't get much fluency. But things are different when you use a full speech signal. If you put a vocalic speech signal in, even if it's not quite matched, you get a bigger improvement in fluency.

Sheena Reilly
If there are conversational treatment effects, whatever their nature and size, what do you think is the likelihood of long-term relapse with these devices?

Tim Saltuklaroglu
Surely a pressing issue. I would suspect that, just like any other treatment for stuttering, we would see some relapse. Perhaps it depends on whether clients need to attend to the signal constantly or whether any effects are a spontaneous adaptation to the AAF signal. Again, this issue requires research. Perhaps the configuration of frequency shift and delay parameters will influence long-term outcome.

Sheena Reilly
You seem not accepting of the Pollard et al. (2009) clinical trial incorporating everyday speech, which appeared to suggest overall that the device will not work for stuttering clients. Can you expand on those concerns?

Tim Saltuklaroglu
I had a problem with that study because of how they defined stuttering. They used a definition of stuttering that included things they taught in their protocol. Consequently, it was difficult to know what was stuttering and what was something they actually taught. Also, to test devices in the real world you need participants to be compliant. Many of the participants in that trial were not really using the device and some lost their devices.

Anne Packman
We were interested in the age range of clients for which you would recommend an AAF device such as SpeechEasy. There is a clip on YouTube of young children being fitted.[3] What is your view about that?

Tim Saltuklaroglu
I have been asked about that a couple of times and I am always conservative with AAF and young children. The youngest child I ever fitted personally was 7 years old and I regret doing that. With that age there are issues with care for the device, being able to attend to the signal, and most importantly, using

[3] http://www.youtube.com/watch?v=Mdc2pT7zTas&feature=related

them in schools. Schools are noisy places and the background noise can be horrendous. I try now to not recommend them for anyone younger than 12 or 13 years. Some people do fit younger children, but I don't. It makes inherent sense in some ways to fit young children because they do tend to respond quite well to AAF. And children generally do not have as many psychological issues as stuttering adults. Given the choice though, I would rather try some other treatment approaches first.

Anne Packman

The brain is more 'plastic' with children, so in theory our group considered that generalisation of any effects may occur better than for adults.

Tim Saltuklaroglu

I agree. And I think research may find easier ways to deliver the feedback for children in their everyday environments. Costs would of course be an issue. The SpeechEasy devices are currently $5000 in the United States and for any parent to send a child to school with this device poses some practical challenges.

Joseph Attanasio

You just mentioned cost. Would that be a potential confound for any clinical trials research. Clearly you place some stock in self-report clinical data. But if a client invests $5000 in a device, is that person about to admit it's not working? Is it the opposite of buyer's remorse? Do you have any information about why the clients make their self-report about the value of these devices?

Tim Saltuklaroglu

It would be difficult to separate out any of those effects. At Eastern Carolina University during the early years of testing, clients received their devices for a nominal cost. We did send a questionnaire survey of people who had bought the devices for full price. I think there is general bias if you ask clients how their treatment went, because they have invested much responsibility in making it work – but this applies to all therapies. So obviously, all this highlights the advantages of objective stuttering count data from blinded observers.

Sheena Reilly

How do you decide in what ear to put the device. Does it make a difference? And does it work differently? We discussed this a lot in relation to brain function.

Tim Saltuklaroglu

In relation to the brain it doesn't matter, because auditory information from both ears goes to both sides of the brain. Assuming normal hearing in both ears, right-handed clients typically choose the right and hold the phone to the left ear so they can use the phone and receive AAF. Also, in terms of manual dexterity, if you are right handed it is easier to put the device in the right ear. If there is a hearing impairment in one ear, you need to work with an audiologist when fitting the device.

Anne Packman

Talking of the brain, we had a brief discussion about mirror neurons and I understand your theoretical support for the use of altered word feedback is that they engage mirror neurons. I believe there is some controversy these days about the actual existence of mirror neurons (de Zubicaray et al., 2010), so would you like to comment about that?

Tim Saltuklaroglu

Certainly, we could debate all day about the existence or lack thereof of a 'mirror system'. For this reason I only alluded to the 'possibility of the mirror system' with a recent reference for its involvement in speech perception (Tremblay and Small, 2011). It is likely a semantic argument to some extent and not intended to be a topic of debate in the present forum. I believe the important message to convey is the link between speech perception and production is well established and it is possible that this link may play a role in aiding fluency in PWS.

References

Antipova, E. A., Purdy, S. C., Blakeley, M., & Williams, S. (2008) Effects of altered auditory feedback (AAF) on stuttering frequency during monologue speech production. *Journal of Fluency Disorders, 33*, 274-290.

Armson, J., & Kalinowski, J. (1994) Interpreting results of the fluent speech paradigm in stuttering research: difficulties in separating cause from effect. *Journal of Speech and Hearing Research, 37*, 69-82.

Chase, R. A., Sutton, S., & Rappin, I. (1961) Sensory feedback influences on motor performance. *Journal of Auditory Research, 1*, 212-213.

Cook, M. J., & Smith, L. M. (2006) Outcomes for adult males using the SpeechEasy® fluency device for one year. Poster presented at the annual convention of the American Speech-Language-Hearing Association, Miami, FL; November.

Dayalu, V. N., Guntupalli, V. K., Kalinowski, J., Stuart, A., Saltuklaroglu, T., & Rastatter, M. P. (2011) Effect of continuous speech and non-speech signals on stuttering frequency in adults who stutter. *Logopedia Phoniatrics Vocology, 36*(3), 121-127.

de Zubicaray, G., Postle, N., McMahon, K., Meredith, M., & Ashton, R. (2010) Mirror neurons, the representation of word meaning, and the foot of the third left frontal convolution. *Brain and Language, 112*, 77-84.

Fox, P. T., Ingham, R. J., Ingham, J. C., Hirsch, T. B., Downs, J. H., Martin, C., & Lancaster, J. L. (1996) A PET study of the neural systems of stuttering. *Nature, 382*, 158-161.

Goldiamond, I. (1965) Stuttering and fluency as manipulatable operant classes. In: L. Krasner & L. P. Ullmann (Eds.), *Research in Behavior Modification*. New York: Holt, Rinehart & Winston.

Hargrave, S., Kalinowski, J., Stuart, A., Armson, J., & Jones, K. (1994) Effect of frequency-altered feedback on stuttering frequency at normal and fast speech rates. *Journal of Speech and Hearing Research, 37*, 1313-1319.

Howell, P., El-Yaniv, N., & Powell, D. J. (1987) Factors affecting fluency in stutterers. In: H. F. M. Peters and W. Hulstijn (Eds.), *Speech Motor Dynamics in Stuttering* (pp. 361-369). New York: Springer Verlag.

Ingham, J. C., 1993, Current status of stuttering and behavior modification: Recent trends in the application of behavior modification in children and adults. *Journal of Fluency Disorders, 18*, 27–55.

Kalinowski, J., Dayalu, V. N., Stuart, A., Rastatter, M. P., & Rami, M. K. (2000) Stutter-free and stutter-filled speech signals and their role in stuttering amelioration for English speaking adults. *Neuroscience Letters, 281*, 198–200.

Kalinowski, J., Guntupalli, V. K., Stuart, A., & Saltuklaroglu, T. (2004) Self-reported efficacy of an ear-level prosthetic device that delivers altered auditory feedback for the management of stuttering. *International Journal of Rehabilitation Research, 27*, 167–170.

Kalinowski, J., & Saltuklaroglu, T. (2003) Choral speech: the amelioration of stuttering via imitation and the mirror neuronal system. *Neuroscience and Biobehavioral Reviews, 27*, 339–347.

Kalinowski, J., & Saltuklaroglu, T. (2006) *Stuttering.* San Diego: Plural Publishing.

Kalinowski, J., & Stuart, A. (1996) Stuttering amelioration at various auditory feedback delays and speech rates. *European Journal of Disorders of Communication, 31*, 259–269.

Lee, B. S. (1951) Artificial stutterer. *Journal of Speech and Hearing Disorders, 16*, 53–55

Lincoln, M., Onslow, M., Packman, A., & Jones, M. (2010) An experimental investigation of the effect of AAF on the conversational speech of adults who stutter. *Journal of Speech, Language and Hearing Research, 53*, 1122–1131.

Lincoln, M., Packman, A., & Onslow, M. (2006) Altered auditory feedback and the treatment of stuttering: A review. *Journal of Fluency Disorders, 31*, 71–79.

Lincoln, M., Packman, A., Onslow, M., & Jones, M. (2010) An experimental investigation of the effect of AAF on the conversational speech of adults who stutter. *Journal of Speech, Language, and Hearing Research, 53*, 1122–1131.

Max, L., Guenther, F. H., Gracco, V. L., Ghosh, S. S., & Wallace, M. E. (2004) Unstable or insufficiently activated internal models and feedback-biased motor control as sources of dysfluency: A theoretical model of stuttering. *Contemporary Issues in Communication Science and Disorders, 31*, 105–122.

Molt, L. (2006) SpeechEasy® AAF device long-term clinical trial: Attitudinal / Perceptual measures. Poster presented at the annual convention of the American Speech-Language-Hearing Association, Miami, FL; November.

Pollard, R., Ellis, J. B., Finan, D., & Ramig, P. R. (2009) Effects of the SpeechEasy on objective and perceived aspects of stuttering: a 6-month, phase I clinical trial in naturalistic environments. *Journal of Speech, Language, and Hearing Research, 52*, 516–533.

Robey, R. R. (2004) A five-phase model for clinical-outcome research. *Journal of Communication Disorders, 37*, 401–411.

Runyan, C. M., Runyan, S. E., & Hibbard, S. (2006). The SpeechEasy device: A three-year study. Poster presented at the annual convention of the American Speech-Language-Hearing Association, Miami, FL; November.

Saltuklaroglu, T., Kalinowski, J., Robbins, M., Crawcour, S., & Bowers, A. (2009) Comparisons of stuttering frequency during and after speech initiation in unaltered feedback, altered auditory feedback and choral speech conditions. *International Journal of Language and Communication Disorders, 44*, 1000–1017.

Saltuklaroglu, T., Kalinowski, J., & Stuart, A. (2010) Refutation of a therapeutic alternative? A reply to Pollard, Ellis, Finan, and Ramig. *Journal of Speech, Language, and Hearing Research, 53*, 908–911.

Stuart, A., Frazier, C. L., Kalinowski, J., & Vos, P. W. (2008) The effect of frequency altered feedback on stuttering duration and type. *Journal of Speech, Language, and Hearing Research, 51*, 889–897.

Stuart, A., & Kalinowski, J. (2004) The perception of speech naturalness of post-therapeutic and altered auditory feedback speech of adults with mild and severe stuttering. *Folia Phoniatrica et Logopaedia, 56*, 347–357.

Stuart, A., Kalinowski, J., Rastatter, M. P., & Lynch, K. (2002) Effect of delayed auditory feedback on normal speakers at two speech rates. *The Journal of the Acoustical Society of America, 111*, 2237–2241.

Stuart, A., Kalinowski, J., Saltuklaroglu, T., & Guntupalli, V. K. (2006) Investigations of the impact of altered auditory feedback in-the-ear devices on the speech of people who stutter: one-year follow-up. *Disability and Rehabilitation, 28*, 757–765.

Tremblay, P., & Small, S. L. (2011) On the context-dependent nature of the contribution of the ventral premotor cortex to speech perception. *Neuroimage, 57*, 1561–1571.

Van Borsel, J., Reunes, G., & Van den Bergh, N. (2003) Delayed auditory feedback in the treatment of stuttering: clients as consumers. *International Journal of Language and Communication Disorders, 38*, 119–129.

Chapter 4
The Lidcombe Program

Rosemarie Hayhow
Speech & Language Therapy Research Unit, Bristol, UK

Overview

The Lidcombe Program (LP) is a parent implemented behavioural treatment for early stuttering (Onslow et al., 2003), designed for children younger than 6 years. The goal of Stage 1 is to attain stutter-free speech or speech with extremely mild stuttering in all situations. The goal of Stage 2 is to maintain this progress in the long term. The parents do the treatment in the child's everyday speaking environment and so training the parents to do this safely and effectively is a crucial part of the clinician's role. There is an international Lidcombe Program Trainers Consortium (http://sydney.edu.au/health_sciences/asrc/health_professionals/lptc.shtml) designed to provide consistent, worldwide training and a freely available treatment guide (Packman et al., 2011).

The primary treatment components are parental verbal contingencies and measurement. Parents provide verbal contingencies for their child's stutter-free speech and less frequent contingencies for unambiguous stuttering. The verbal contingencies for stutter-free speech are acknowledgement, praise and requests for self-evaluation. The verbal contingencies for unambiguous stuttering are acknowledgement and requests for self-correction. Parents use a 10-point severity rating scale to record their child's daily severity of stuttering. The scale is 1 = no stuttering, 2 = extremely mild stuttering and 10 = extremely severe stuttering. Parents are taught how to use this scale and the clinician checks the consistency of their ratings each week. This is necessary so that the severity ratings give a reliable indication of progress and can be used by the clinician and parent to guide treatment decisions about how the treatment should change over time. The clinician counts moments of stuttering in a clinic speech sample of around 300 syllables at the beginning of each clinic visit. The severity ratings and percent syllables stuttered (%SS) are used to

The Science and Practice of Stuttering Treatment: A Symposium, First Edition. Edited by Suzana Jelčić Jakšić and Mark Onslow.

determine the child's readiness for the transition from Stage 1 to Stage 2 and the completion of treatment.[1]

During Stage 1 the parent and child attend weekly 1-hour clinic sessions. This is when parents learn how to provide verbal contingencies. First, they learn to give verbal contingencies during structured conversations, by altering the nature of the conversation with their child to achieve predominantly stutter-free speaking. This is done by selecting topics and materials, and by using conversational strategies that result in low levels of stuttering. For example, in the early days of treatment parents may select activities that use visual materials and may modify their own speaking so that the child can respond with relatively short utterances. Parents engage their children in one or two short structured talking times each day so that parents can give contingencies for stutter-free speech with only the occasional request for self-correction when stuttering occurs. Parents learn how to do this from the demonstration and guidance of the clinician.

As parent severity ratings reduce, showing that treatment is having an effect, the parent learns to give verbal contingencies during everyday conversations that occur naturally between parent and child. With continued progress the number of structured conversations are systematically reduced until all or nearly all treatment is given during everyday, unstructured conversations.

The treatment components of measurement and verbal contingencies are the same for all children, but the way they are presented to each child is individualised. Many children are happy with the verbal contingencies but some are more sensitive to any parental feedback and so the frequency and style of verbal contingencies will vary accordingly. However, the overriding consideration is that there needs to be a balance between the verbal contingencies being sufficient for a treatment effect but not feeling invasive for a child.

Benchmarks are available for clinical progress. Clinicians can expect a reduction in severity ratings by one-third after five clinic visits (Onslow et al., 2002) and a median of 14 clinic visits is required to reach the criteria for completion of Stage 1. There are four retrospective file audit studies ($N = 591$) from which the latter benchmark is derived showing remarkably consistent results (Jones et al., 2000; Kingston et al., 2003; Koushik et al., 2011; Onslow et al., 2002).

Theoretical basis

The LP did not derive from a particular causal theory of stuttering. It is an empirically based treatment that drew upon empirical laboratory findings for

[1]Members of the Lidcombe Program Trainers' Consortium met in Philadelphia in November 2010. One agenda item was discussion of the removal of %SS as a mandatory component of the treatment. The Consortium decided to make this change and the current version of the treatment guide outlines the new procedures (Packman et al., 2011). The rationale for the change is outlined in Bridgman et al. (2011).

its development. It was found, in the laboratory context, that stuttering could be reduced by verbal contingencies in preschool children (Martin et al., 1972; Reed and Godden, 1977; for a review, see Onslow, 2003). The LP development was driven by the need to find ways for parents to present verbal stimulation to their stuttering children during everyday life.

Demonstrated value

The research evidence for the LP with preschool-age children – children younger than 6 years – will be considered with reference to the well-known Phase I–Phase III clinical trials development sequence described by Pocock (1983). For present purposes, the Onslow et al. (2008) definition of a stuttering clinical trial is applied: a prospective attempt to determine the efficacy of an entire treatment with at least 3-months follow-up, and speech observations beyond the clinic. Phase I and II clinical trials determine whether a treatment might work as expected, with no harmful or unwanted effects, on a small number of cases. During the 1990s, two such small-scale trials, both non-randomised, provided evidence to support further LP clinical trials development (Onslow et al., 1990, 1994[2]). Woods et al. (2002) showed that these results were not accompanied by any adverse psychological reaction from children. An additional, non-randomised clinical trial was reported during the following decade by Rousseau et al. (2007). There was an independent replication by Miller and Guitar (2009) using a follow-up design of cases previously treated.

A Phase III randomised controlled trial was reported by Jones et al. (2005) and the successful results of that trial were replicated with a similar design by Lattermann et al. (2008), although the latter report was not a clinical trial according to the Onslow et al. (2008) definition because it involved only 16 weeks of LP treatment. Long-term follow-up of cases from clinical trials (Jones et al., 2008; Lincoln and Onslow, 1997) and retrospective file audits (Koushik et al., 2011) suggest that treatment effects are durable, although Jones et al. (2008) reported that relapse can occur after children attain stutter-free speech. In that report 19 children were followed up at a mean of 5 years post-treatment and three were found to be stuttering above 1.0 %SS when telephoned unexpectedly.

A recent meta-analysis was conducted for 134 children who received the LP in randomised controlled trials or randomised controlled experiments (Onslow et al., 2012). Results showed an odds ratio of 7.5, meaning that children who received the entire LP or a portion of it were 7.5 times more likely to have stuttering below 1.0 %SS than children who received no treatment. Results are summarised in Figure 4.1.

[2]The protocol of the Onslow et al. (1994) report was a randomised controlled trial, however, the children could not be retained in the control group so the results are presented here as a Phase II trial.

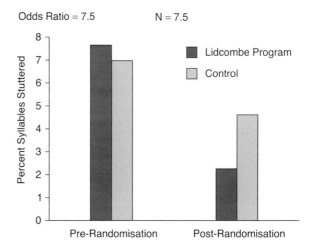

Figure 4.1 Results of a meta-analysis of children who were in randomised controlled trials and experiments with the Lidcombe Program (LP).

Advantages and disadvantages

Advantages

In relation to other early stuttering interventions, the evidence base for the LP is generally acknowledged as strong, and with more evidence to support its use than any other early intervention (Bloodstein and Bernstein Ratner, 2008; Bothe et al., 2006; Kalinowski and Saltuklaroglu, 2006; Yairi and Ambrose, 2005). Two qualitative studies report positive experiences by parents who use the LP. Goodhue et al. (2010) reported maternal experience of increased quality time with their stuttering children and improved parenting skills during the course of treatment. Mothers also reported increased knowledge of stuttering and its management as a benefit of the programme. Parents reported that their children enjoyed the verbal contingency procedures and the clinic visits.

Hayhow (2009) reported that when children made steady progress, mothers found using the LP with their children straightforward, and some expressed surprise that such simple procedures could have such a positive effect. These parents were enthusiastic and innovative with a capacity for independent problem solving. However, Hayhow reported a group of parents for whom treatment progress was initially straightforward, and then the treatment process became somewhat problematic. Hayhow also reported a minority of parents whose treatment was difficult from the outset. These parents found the verbal contingencies difficult to manage, experienced problems in leading the child through activities and did not develop the problem-solving skills that were apparent in the straightforward group. These parents held some beliefs about childhood stuttering that made the treatment problematic for them.

Clinicians have reported that the LP encourages an open attitude towards stuttering in both parents and children who nearly always become more comfortable about stuttering (Hayhow, 2005). The same clinicians also reported that they and many parents liked being actively involved in treatment, and felt empowered by knowing specifically how to handle the problem. This could be linked to treatment happening where stuttering occurs, during everyday conversations. It may also be linked to the fact that the LP in no way implicates parents in the cause of stuttering or its perpetuation. Stuttering reduction without altered speech patterns is arguably one of the advantages of the LP (Hayhow, 2011).

Disadvantages

There are several components of the LP specified in the treatment guide (Packman et al., 2011) and it is unknown, which of them are essential to any treatment effects and which are not. At present there is only sketchy and preliminary evidence about the matter. Harrison et al. (2004) provided some suggestion that the verbal contingencies for stuttered speech might be essential and that parent severity ratings might not. Koushik et al. (2011) provided preliminary evidence that clinic visits each week might not be essential. The Lidcombe Program Trainers Consortium deliberated about whether clinicians measuring %SS within the clinic was an essential treatment component, and decided it was not (Bridgman et al., 2011; see Footnote p. 44).

At present no mechanism is known for why the LP might work. Although the LP is not driven by causal theory, as described previously, that of course does not stop speculation about the mechanisms by which it might be able to control early stuttering. At present, those mechanisms are unknown, with some evidence that post-treatment acoustic changes are not responsible (Onslow et al., 2002), and some evidence that frank change of children's language function is not involved either (Bonelli et al., 2000; Lattermann et al., 2005). There is some suggestion that the LP may facilitate whatever mechanism might be responsible for natural recovery (O'Brian and Onslow, 2011).

During the period of its development, understanding of possible causal factors for stuttering has increased. There is now evidence of subtle differences in brain structure (e.g. Brown et al., 2005; Sommer et al., 2002) and evidence of differences in brain functioning affecting speech motor control (Alm, 2004; Packman et al., 2007; Smith et al., 2010). Those differences appear to exist with school-age children who stutter (Chang et al., 2008). Should those differences be involved with stuttering causality, speculation is possible that children might learn a 'work-around for that neuroanatomical problem' (Onslow and Yaruss 2007, p. 67). Indeed, a constructivist view of the matter is that children are actively engaged in making sense of their experiences (Butler and Green 2007). From this perspective, requests for self-correction provide a protected space within a conversation where children can experiment with more effective ways of managing their moments of stuttering, which cannot be done during usual childhood conversation. Bernstein Ratner and Guitar (2006) discuss a range of effects that the LP might have on parents, such as reducing anxiety about stuttering and providing supportive speech attention. These are among many potential explanations for documented treatment effects that might attribute them to factors other than, or in addition to, the verbal contingencies.

The LP has been associated with potential negative parent experiences. Goodhue et al. (2010) and Hayhow (2009) reported that parents could experience guilt because of feeling that they are not doing the treatment properly. Hayhow specifically sought a group of parents for whom treatment was not proceeding satisfactorily, and found certain associated case history features. These included a strong family history of stuttering, other speech and language problems, learning difficulties or co-morbid diagnoses of dyspraxia or other motor problems. Such parents require more support when treatment takes longer.

Children as young as 2 years may be aware of their stuttering and some may be distressed by it (Boey et al. 2009). Preschool children may suffer negative social consequences when they stutter in front of their peers (Langevin et al., 2009). However, there is some evidence that LP treatment might not be as suitable for younger children as it is for older children (Jones et al., 2000; Kingston et al., 2003) and so there is a tension between allowing time for natural recovery to take its course and protecting children from potentially harmful peer responses and negative self-evaluation.

Conclusions and future directions

The LP has come a long way since its early development by Onslow and colleagues in Sydney. It is now widely used in many countries and there is an increasing evidence base. Quantitative studies have helped to establish its effectiveness and safety and qualitative studies have helped us understand more of the experiences of the parents and clinicians who use the programme. Future research may help us work more effectively with challenging cases and continued refinement of the treatment should ensure that the programme remains a viable treatment option in the future.

Current and future developments of the LP are geared to improve access to the treatment by increasing its availability and its clinical efficiency. With regards to the former, a series of trials of the treatment in telehealth format provides potential for it to reach families who have no local services or who are unable to attend their nearest clinic (Harrison et al., 1999; Lewis et al., 2008; Wilson et al., 2004). Results generally show that such a treatment format requires twice as long for the completion of Stage 1, however current developments of webcam technology might be expected to improve that situation. A randomised controlled trial of the LP with in-clinic presentation and webcam presentation is currently being investigated. The trial is a collaboration between La Trobe University in Melbourne, Australia, and the Australian

Stuttering Research Centre in Sydney, Australia. Such developments might eventually lead to a useful stepped care model of early intervention.[3] With regards to treatment efficiency, a randomised controlled clinical trial of group treatment has been completed (Lees et al., 2011). The collaborating centres for that trial are the same as for the webcam trial mentioned previously.

With regards to increasing clinical efficiency there is much to learn about what parents actually do in home treatment and in trying to establish which aspects of the programme are essential for progress. A preliminary study of what parents actually do has been published (Carr-Swift et al., 2011). Mixed method studies may add to our understanding of the essential treatment components (Hayhow, 2011) and so lead to more efficient treatment.

Finally, an international translational research programme of the LP is under way in Australia, North America and the United Kingdom, for the purpose of determining to what extent community clinicians can match the results that have been attained in clinical trials. The first results from the Australian part of that research have been completed (O'Brian et al., 2011) and at the time of writing, a paper based on those results is in peer review.

Discussion

Sheena Reilly

A critical issue our group came up with is whether there is any danger if parents request self-corrections of the wrong behaviours, if they use verbal contingencies for stutter-free speech?

Rosemarie Hayhow

It can happen of course if they mistake stutter-free speech for stuttering. It is more likely to happen when the treatment starts to be successful and parents focus on normal disfluencies. What often happens, in my experience, is that parents will say 'I've noticed he has started saying whole words a couple of times' when in fact there is no reason to think that might be stuttering. But then parents often say, 'but I started looking at other children and I've noticed they're doing it too'. This is one of the reasons why the LP instructs parents only to use verbal contingencies for unambiguous stuttering and to ignore speech events when there is any doubt. As we say during Lidcombe Program Trainers Consortium teaching, 'if in doubt, leave it out'.

Sheena Reilly

Would the clinician ensure that parents do this correctly?

[3]The Stepped Care model of health care delivery contains two fundamentals (Bower and Gilbody, 2005). It provides the simplest and most cost efficient method of health care that is efficacious. It is self-correcting so that patients progressively escalate to more resource intensive, and less cost efficient, model health care if they are shown to need it. It is suitable for disorders where simple, cost efficient interventions can be used for a significant proportion of those affected. A similar model, specifically developed for early stuttering management is described by Hayhow (2007).

Rosemarie Hayhow

Yes, absolutely. The treatment guide specifies that at each clinic visit parents demonstrate to the clinician how they have been presenting the verbal contingencies. So the clinician does watch the process closely. We never ask parents to do things that we don't see them do in the clinic first. If parents were making any errors with their requests for self-correction, or any other verbal contingencies, a clinician would be expected to pick that up.

Ann Packman

Our primary question is why does it work? You presented various alternatives, but what do you think?

Rosemarie Hayhow

Of course we don't know at present. As we say during Lidcombe Program Trainers Consortium teaching, one explanation is that the verbal contingencies provide stimulus control. But that really is not a deep explanation neither is what I said about providing a safe environment in which a child can experiment with dealing with their moments of stuttering. That can't happen in everyday conversation, but when we say 'would you like to smooth that out' it encourages children to find their own way of dealing with it. We certainly are not telling them to change their speech pattern or to slow down. Preschoolers have some neural plasticity remaining with speech motor development, and perhaps the treatment capitalises on that. By encouraging children to self-correct we are reducing the opportunities for practising stuttering, this may also be an important factor.

Joseph Attanasio

You said the LP is not based on a putative cause of stuttering itself. Perhaps it is based on motor learning theory?

Rosemarie Hayhow

It was not based on motor learning theory, but that might explain why it works. It certainly works differently from the indirect treatment for preschoolers we will hear about and discuss tomorrow (see Chapter 13). I think there is a difference, a very important difference. With the LP we are inviting children to learn how to deal with these little glitches that are happening in their speaking and so we are encouraging them to take a very active role in the management of that problem, rather than hoping that by creating a facilitating environment the child will develop through a period of stuttering. Feedback plays an important role in motor learning and parental contingencies provide the children with specific feedback. This feedback helps them distinguish between stuttered and stutter-free speech. Initially, during the talk-times, parents give frequent contingencies but then as treatment progress the children increasingly rely upon their internal feedback mechanisms. This process of a gradual shift from external to internal feedback is consistent with motor learning theory.

Ann Packman

I have an interesting question for you from the group. Why after so long and with so much evidence, is there still so much controversy about the LP.

Rosemarie Hayhow

I don't understand it. I think many still see the LP as a cold programme, and I don't think that idea goes away until clinicians have Lidcombe Program Consortium training and discover that it is a supportive and child-centred treatment. It may also be the case that indirect treatments are based on complex models of what causes early stuttering, and there are many who believe those models to be correct and that a complex problem requires complex assessment and treatment. I suppose it is a different way of thinking about early stuttering, that it can be managed by something as simple as verbal contingencies, I also think behavioural treatments got a bad reputation around the 1970s and they were seen as taking a limited view of the problem, as clinically 'cold' and not suitable for small children. But the Goodhue et al. (2010) and Hayhow (2009) studies indicate this not necessarily the case for the LP. These reports also show that things don't go well for parents if the treatment is not going so well, but that would be expected for any treatment.

Sheena Reilly

My group was interested in any comments you can make on the characteristics of children that you wouldn't use the LP with, and if so what were they like? And are there any predictors of which children do better? We talked about possible factors such as age of the child, the type of family and temperamental characteristics.

Rosemarie Hayhow

The Jones et al. (2000) and Kingston et al. (2003) file audit reports showed that little could predict how long Stage 1 treatment took. More severe stuttering pre-treatment was related to slightly longer treatment times, and very young children shortly after onset also required more clinic visits. That was intuitive to us because the LP makes cognitive demands of children. Now there are clinical trials data about an even simpler treatment that would be suitable for very young children, that gives an alternative to consider in those situations (see Chapter 15). I am now participating with colleagues from Australia and the United Kingdom in the translational research I mentioned. That research is designed to determine features of children and parents – such as their psychological and temperament status – clinician training and clinical workplaces that might impact on how well the treatment goes. From a clinically anecdotal viewpoint, a number of factors recur for us. Children who have additional speech and language problems, a very strong family history of stuttering, dyspraxia and learning difficulties are going to take longer and may not achieve low levels of stuttering. Another problem group is children who have stuttering and cluttering, where a reduction in frequency and severity of stuttering often occurs but residual rapid syllable repetitions persist. Otherwise most children seem to do well. Please note though that I am discussing children younger than 6 years, which is the age group for whom the treatment was developed; see Chapter 5 for the Lidcombe Program with school-age children.

Joseph Attanasio

Could you carry on with this discussion to include cultural and multi-cultural issues, parent/clinician culture and culture in general. Do cultural issues ever impair the treatment?

Rosemarie Hayhow

This is so complex. The client population we have in Bristol has many refugee families from different parts of Africa and there are all sorts of reasons why doing something like the LP is difficult with them. I think you need to assess each case on its own merits. I would never want to disregard the LP as an option with a family because they are in difficult circumstances or come from a different cultural background. Some of them have done extremely well. But always we are on the lookout for LP features that are culturally difficult for families, and for those families who have other problems going on at the same time. Margaret Weber, who retired from the Lidcombe Program Trainers Consortium some years ago, used to say, 'assume nothing', which I think was good advice. Incidentally, we begin Consortium training by pointing out that clinical trials have shown effects for children all over the world. This includes European countries such as Germany, as well as countries like Iran whose language and culture differ markedly from the Western countries where the programme was developed.

Sheena Reilly

Is the LP the same for each child and parent?

Rosemarie Hayhow

Yes. In as much as the contingencies and the severity ratings are the same. However, for each child and parent the presentation of those standard features will differ. Verbal contingencies during structured conversation will be different from one child to the next because we follow the child's interests and personality as much as we can. And verbal contingencies during everyday conversations will always differ between parent-child pairs. That is one of the fundamentals of the treatment: the clinician needs to find a way to make measurement and verbal contingencies work in a unique way for every family.

Ann Packman

Another question from our group was at what point would you move on if a child wasn't achieving the desired target and what would you do move on to a different treatment?

Rosemarie Hayhow

There have been such children, albeit few. If I felt that the LP had achieved as much as it could with a particular child and that there were other things that were standing in the way of the child making further progress then I would address those as best I could with the skills that I have and I think that's all I have time to say.

Joseph Attanasio

Rosemarie you mentioned that, or you hinted, that there might be non-essential components to the LP. Could you clarify them and tell us what they might be?

Rosemarie Hayhow

I don't really want to go further than the Harrison et al. (2004) and Koushik et al. (2011) reports I mentioned that raised some prospect that verbal contingencies for stuttered speech may be important, that parent severity ratings may not and that the weekly visit to the clinic may not be optimal. I cannot imagine doing the programme without the severity ratings and wonder whether their lack of importance in Harrison's study was because she looked only at the first 4 weeks of treatment. As time goes on, many parents use severity ratings in an almost intuitive way to help them decide upon the level of structure for home treatment. Without the severity ratings parents might struggle to make these judgments based on subtle changes in their children's hour-to-hour and day-to-day talking. They are also a tool for communication between parent and clinician. However, we need to wait until we have enough data to continue to pare things back as we did with in-clinic %SS in the Bridgman et al. (2011) paper and to keep an open mind with regards to improving the treatment experience for children and their parents.

References

Alm, P. (2004) Stuttering and the basal ganglia circuits: a critical review of possible relations. *Journal of Communication Disorders, 37*, 325-369.

Bernstein Ratner, N., & Guitar, B. (2006) Treatment of very early stuttering and parent-administered therapy: The state of the art. In: N. Bernstein Ratner & J. Tetnowski (Eds.), *Current Issues in Stuttering Research and Practice* (pp. 99-124). Mahwah, NJ: Lawrence Erlbaum Associates.

Bloodstein, O., & Bernstein Ratner, N. (2008) *A Handbook on Stuttering.* Clifton Park, NY: Delmar.

Boey, R., Van de Heyning, P., Wuyts, F., Heylen, L., Stoop, R., & De Bodt, M. (2009) Awareness and reactions of young stuttering children aged 2-7 years old towards their speech disfluency. *Journal of Communication Disorders, 42*, 334-346.

Bonelli, P., Dixon, M., Bernstein Ratner, N., & Onslow, M. (2000) Child and parent speech and language following the Lidcombe Program of early stuttering intervention. *Clinical Linguistics and Phonetics, 14*, 427-446.

Bothe, A. K., Davidow, J. H., Bramlett, R. E., & Ingham, R. J. (2006) Stuttering treatment research 1970-2005: I. Systematic review incorporating trial quality assessment of behavioral, cognitive, and related approaches. *American Journal of Speech-Language Pathology, 15*, 321-341.

Bower, P., & Gilbody, S. (2005) Stepped care in psychological therapies: access, effectiveness, and efficiency. *British Journal of Psychiatry, 186*, 11-17.

Bridgman, K., Onslow, M., O'Brian, S., Block, S., & Jones, M. (2011) Changes to stuttering measurement during the Lidcombe Program treatment process. *Asia Pacific Journal of Speech, Language, and Hearing, 14*, 147-152.

Brown, S., Ingham, R., Ingham, J., Laird, A., & Fox, P. (2005) Stuttered and fluent speech production: An ALE meta-analysis of functional neuroimaging studies. *Human Brain Mapping, 25*, 105-117.

Butler, R., & Green, D. (2007) *The Child Within.* Chichester, UK: Wiley.

Carr-Swift, M., O'Brian, S., Hewat, S., Onslow, M., Packman, A., & Menzies, R. (2011) Investigating parent treatment in the Lidcombe Program: Three case studies. *International Journal of Speech-Language Pathology, 13*, 308-316.

Chang, S. E., Erickson, K. I., Ambrose, N. G., Hasegawa-Johnson, M. A., & Ludlow, C. L. (2008) Brain anatomy differences in childhood stuttering. *NeuroImage, 39*, 1333-1344.

Goodhue, R., Onslow, M., Quine, S., O'Brian, S., & Hearne, A. (2010) The Lidcombe Program of early stuttering intervention: Mothers' experiences. *Journal of Fluency Disorders, 35*, 70-84.

Harrison, E., Onslow, M., & Menzies, R. (2004) Dismantling the Lidcombe Program of early stuttering intervention: Verbal contingencies for stuttering and clinical measurement. *International Journal of Language and Communication Disorders, 39*, 257-267.

Harrison, E., Wilson, L., & Onslow, M. (1999) Distance intervention for early stuttering with the Lidcombe Programme. *Advances in Speech Language Pathology, 1*, 31-36.

Hayhow, R. (2005) An exploration of speech & language therapists' experience of using the Lidcombe Program. Paper presented at the 7th Oxford Dysfluency Conference, Oxford, UK.

Hayhow, R. (2007) The least first framework. In: S. Roulstone (Ed.), *Prioritising Child Health: Practice and Principles.* London: Routledge.

Hayhow, R. (2009) Parents' experiences of the Lidcombe Program of early stuttering intervention. *International Journal of Speech-Language Pathology, 11*, 20-25.

Hayhow, R. (2011) Does it work? Why does it work? Reconciling difficult questions. *International Journal of Language and Communication Disorders, 46*, 155-168

Jones, M., Hearne, A., Onslow, M., Ormond, T., Williams, S., Schwarz, I., & O'Brian, S. (2008) Extended follow up of a randomised controlled trial of the Lidcombe Program of Early Stuttering Intervention. *International Journal of Language and Communication Disorders, 7*, 1-13.

Jones, M., Onslow, M., Harrison, E., & Packman, A. (2000) Treating stuttering in young children: Predicting treatment time in the Lidcombe Program. *Journal of Speech, Language, and Hearing Research, 43*, 1440-1450.

Jones, M., Onslow, M., Packman, A., Williams, S., Ormond, T., Schwarz, I., & Gebski, V. (2005) Randomised controlled trial of the Lidcombe programme of early stuttering intervention. *British Medical Journal, 331*, 659-661.

Kalinowski, J. S., & Saltuklaroglu, T. (2006) *Stuttering.* San Diego, CA: Plural Publishing.

Kingston, M., Huber, A., Onslow, M., Jones, M., & Packman, A. (2003) Predicting treatment time in the Lidcombe Program: Replication and meta-analysis. *International Journal of Language and Communication Disorders, 38*, 165-177.

Koushik, S., Hewat, S., Shenker, R., Jones, M., & Onslow, M. (2011) North-American Lidcombe Program file audit: Replication and meta-analysis. *International Journal of Language and Communication Disorders, 13*, 301-307.

Langevin, M., Onslow, M., & Packman, A. (2009) Peer responses to stuttering in the preschool setting. *American Journal of Speech-Language Pathology, 18*, 264-276.

Lattermann, C., Euler, H. A., & Neumann, K. (2008) A randomized control trial to investigate the impact of the Lidcombe Program on early stuttering in German-speaking preschoolers. *Journal of Fluency Disorders, 33*, 52-65.

Lattermann, C., Shenker, R. C., & Thordardottir, E. (2005) Progression of language complexity during treatment with the Lidcombe Program for early stuttering intervention. *American Journal of Speech-Language Pathology, 14*, 242-253.

Lees, S., Onslow, M., O'Brian, S., Packman, A., Menzies, R., & Block, S. (2011) Exploring group delivery of the Lidcombe Program of Early Stuttering Intervention from a theoretical perspective. Symposium conducted at the 9th Oxford Dysfluency Conference, Oxford, United Kingdom.

Lewis, C., Onslow, M., Packman, A., Jones, M., & Simpson, J. A. (2008) Phase II trial of telehealth delivery of the Lidcombe Program of early stuttering intervention. *American Journal of Speech-Language Pathology, 17*, 139-149.

Lincoln, M., & Onslow, M. (1997) Long-term outcome of an early intervention for stuttering. *American Journal of Speech-Language Pathology, 6*, 51-58.

Martin, R., Kuhl, P., & Haroldson, S. (1972) An experimental treatment with two preschool stuttering children. *Journal of Speech, Language, and Hearing Research, 15*, 743-752.

Miller, B., & Guitar, B. (2009) Long-term outcome of the Lidcombe Program for early stuttering intervention. *American Journal of Speech-Language Pathology, 18*, 42-49.

O'Brian, S., & Onslow, M. (2011) Clinical management of stuttering children and adults. *British Medical Journal. 342*: d3742.

O'Brian, S., Jones, M., Iverach, L., Onslow, M., Packman, A., & Menzies, R. (2011) *Lidcombe Program Translational Research.* Poster presented at the 9th Oxford Dysfluency Conference, Oxford, United Kingdom; September.

Onslow, M. (2003) From laboratory to living room: The origins and development of the Lidcombe Program. In: M. Onslow, A. Packman & E. Harrison (Eds.), *The Lidcombe Program of Early Stuttering Intervention: A Clinician's Guide* (pp. 21-25). Austin, TX: Pro-ed.

Onslow, M., Andrews, C., & Lincoln, M. (1994) A control-experimental trial of an operant treatment for early stuttering. *Journal of Speech and Hearing Research, 37*, 1244-1259.

Onslow, M., Costa, L., & Rue, S. (1990) Direct early intervention with stuttering: some preliminary data. *Journal of Speech and Hearing Disorders, 55*, 405-416.

Onslow, M., Harrison, E., Jones, M., & Packman, A. (2002) Beyond-clinic speech measures during the Lidcombe Program of early stuttering intervention. *Acquiring Knowledge in Speech, Language and Hearing, 4*, 82-85.

Onslow, M., Jones, M., O'Brian, S., Menzies, R., & Packman, A. (2008). Defining, identifying, and evaluating clinical trials of stuttering treatments: A tutorial for clinicians. *American Journal of Speech-Language Pathology, 17*, 401-415.

Onslow, M., Jones, M., Menzies, R., O'Brian, S., & Packman, A. (2012) Stuttering. In: P. Sturmey & M. Hersen (Eds.), *Handbook of Evidence-Based Practice in Clinical Psychology.* Hoboken, NJ: Wiley.

Onslow, M., Packman, A., & Harrison, E. (Eds.) (2003) *The Lidcombe Program of Early Stuttering Intervention: A Clinician's Guide.* Austin, TX: Pro-ed.

Onslow, M., Stocker, S., Packman, A., & McLeod, S. (2002) Speech segment timing in children after the Lidcombe Program of early stuttering intervention. *Clinical Linguistics and Phonetics, 16*, 21-33.

Onslow, M., & Yaruss, J. S. (2007) Differing perspectives on what to do with a stuttering preschooler and why. *American Journal of Speech-Language Pathology, 16*, 65-68.

Packman, A., Code, C., & Onslow, M. (2007) On the cause of stuttering: Integrating theory with brain and behavioural research. *Journal of Neurolinguistics, 20*, 253-362.

Packman, A., Onslow, M., Webber, M., Harrison, E., Lees, S., Bridgman, K., & Carey, B. (2011) The Lidcombe Program of early stuttering intervention treatment Guide.

Retrieved from http://sydney.edu.au/health_sciences/asrc/health_profession als/asrc_download.shtml

Pocock, S. J. (1983) *Clinical Trials*. Chichester, UK: Wiley.

Reed, C., & Godden, A. (1977) An experimental treatment using verbal punishment with two preschool stutterers. *Journal of Fluency Disorders, 2*, 225–233.

Rousseau, I., Packman, A., Onslow, M., Harrison, L., & Jones, M. (2007) An investigation of language and phonological development and the responsiveness of preschool age children to the Lidcombe Program. *Journal of Communication Disorders, 40*, 382–397.

Smith, A., Sadagopan, N., Walsh, B., & Weber-Fox, C. (2010) Increasing phonological complexity reveals heightened instability in inter-articulatory coordination in adults who stutter. *Journal of Fluency Disorders, 35*, 1–18.

Sommer, M., Koch, M., Paulus, W., Weller, C., & Buchel, C. (2002) Disconnection of speech-relevant brain areas in persistent developmental stuttering. *The Lancet, 360*, 380–383.

Wilson, L., Onslow, M., & Lincoln, M. (2004) Telehealth adaptation of the Lidcombe Program of early stuttering intervention: preliminary data. *American Journal of Speech-Language Pathology, 13*, 81–93.

Woods, S., Shearsby, J., Onslow, M., & Burnham, D. (2002) Psychological impact of the Lidcombe Program of early stuttering intervention. *International Journal of Language and Communication Disorders, 37*, 31–40.

Yairi, E., & Ambrose, N. G. (2005) *Early Childhood Stuttering for Clinicians by Clinicians*. Austin, TX: Pro-Ed.

Chapter 5

Lidcombe Program with School-Age Children

Rosalee C. Shenker[1] and Sarita Koushik[2]

[1]Montreal Fluency Centre, Montreal, QC, Canada
[2]University of Newcastle, Newcastle, Australia and Montreal Fluency Centre,
Westmount, QC, Canada

Overview

Stuttering is most responsive to treatment during the preschool years (Bothe, 2004; Bothe et al., 2006; Ingham and Cordes, 1999; Onslow, 1996; Onslow and Packman, 1999; Prins and Ingham, 1983). Studies indicate that stuttering becomes less responsive to treatment after the preschool years and perhaps more difficult to treat, as a result of the accompanying decrease of neural plasticity (Wohlert and Smith, 2002). It is during this time that demands on communication increase. Children have less access to their parents, live outside the home, become busier and their peer groups become more important. Older children may object to parental help with speaking. Additionally, older children have a longer history of stuttering, and are less likely to recover naturally without treatment. They have limited time for treatment and may have had treatment failures. They are more likely to be bullied, teased or rejected as a result of stuttering. Therefore, the school-age period from 7 to 12 years is an important time of life for receiving an efficacious stuttering treatment.

There have been nine published clinical trials that include school-age children as participants. These trials involve 131 children. Treatments involved include graduated increase in length and complexity of utterance (Ryan and Van Kirk Ryan, 1983, 1995), regulated breathing (de Kindkelder and Boelens, 1998), speech restructuring (see Preface for a definition of this term) (Boberg and Kully, 1994; Budd et al., 1986; Hancock et al., 1998), verbal response contingent stimulation (Lincoln et al., 1996) and electromyographic (EMG) biofeedback (Craig et al., 1996).

There is one failure to replicate EMG biofeedback in a trial for school-age children (Block et al., 2004) (and also a failed replication for adolescents: Huber et al., 2003), and there are no Phase III randomised trials for any of these treatments. For school-age children the strongest evidence is for speech

The Science and Practice of Stuttering Treatment: A Symposium, First Edition. Edited by
Suzana Jelčić Jakšić and Mark Onslow.
© 2012 John Wiley & Sons, Ltd. Published 2012 by John Wiley & Sons, Ltd.

restructuring, with four independent replications and no published failures to replicate. With speech restructuring, clients are taught to use a novel speaking pattern to reduce or eliminate stuttering. Subsequently, speech is shaped to near normal sounding levels and transferred to everyday situations.

While this is a viable format for school-age children, such an approach may not be practical during the busy life of these children. This style of treatment is often based on multiday intensive treatment formats, initially developed for adults and requiring up to 100 treatment hours (Andrews et al., 1980; Onslow et al., 1996). Another issue is the post-treatment relapse that has been reported for this therapy, with estimates between 30% and 50% in clinical trials (Boberg and Kully, 1994; Howie et al., 1981; Martin, 1981; Perkins, 1981).

Could a more simple treatment, such as the Lidcombe Program (LP), be equally effective for school-age children? The LP is a two-stage behavioural treatment that was developed for preschool children (Onslow et al., 2003). In Stage 1, the goal of treatment is to either eliminate stuttering or reduce it to very low levels. Stage 2 is designed to maintain that reduction for a long period. Treatment involves verbal response contingent stimulation that is administered by parents. The clinician supervises that process during weekly clinic visits. The clinician trains the parent to present verbal contingencies for the child's stutter-free speech and unambiguous stuttering. Parents learn to implement those verbal contingencies in structured conversations and in the unstructured conversations of daily living throughout the day in a variety of natural settings. In order to guide the clinical process, the clinician measures percent syllables stuttered (%SS) in the clinic[1] and the parent provides speech measures beyond the clinic. The latter incorporates severity measured on a 10-point perceptual scale. The LP is described in detail in the treatment guide (Packman et al., 2011). Because the LP does not involve the need for a novel speech pattern, it may be a viable treatment for school-age children.

Theoretical basis

There is no consensus about the cause of stuttering. There is, however, an extensive body of evidence that stuttering responds to contingent stimulation (for an overview, see Bloodstein and Bernstein Ratner, 2008) Specifically, there is modest evidence that the stuttering of preschool children is controllable with response contingent stimulation (Martin et al., 1972; Reed and

---

[1]Since the date of the symposium, members of the Lidcombe Program Trainers Consortium met in Philadelphia during November 2010. On the agenda of that meeting was consideration of a growing number of reasons for considering that %SS should be deleted as a mandatory component of the treatment guide. The Consortium decided to make this change and the current version of the treatment guide outlines the new procedures (Packman et al., 2011). The rationale for the treatment is outlined in Bridgman et al. (2011).

Godden, 1977) and modest evidence also that this is the case with school-age children (Martin and Berndt, 1970; Onslow et al., 1997).

The LP was developed independently of any view of stuttering causality. It is a behavioural treatment that was developed empirically from the laboratory findings described previously, rather than from a particular view of the nature of stuttering. The rational for this treatment is based on research that shows stuttering to have operant-like properties and that it may respond to verbal contingencies (Harrison and Onslow, 2009; Packman and Attanasio, 2004).

Demonstrated value

Is the LP viable for children older than 6 years? There are two substantive studies of the LP with school-age children, and one case study. Lincoln et al. (1996) conducted a non-randomised, Phase I trial of the treatment with 11 children ranging in age from 6 years 10 months to 12 years 4 months (median age 7 years 8 months). Speech measures were %SS and speech rate in syllables per minute (SPM) from audio recordings of natural conversational speech samples from a series of measures from 2 months pre-treatment to 12 months post-treatment. A blinded, independent observer made the speech measures. Inter-observer reliability was established with a sample of pre-treatment and post-treatment samples by an independent clinician. A median of twelve 1-hour sessions was required for the children to reduce stuttering to below a mean %SS of 1.5 on measures obtained within and beyond the clinic. Five participants failed to meet programme criteria at some time during the Stage 2 maintenance period, but the majority maintained close to zero stuttering in beyond-clinic contexts at follow-up at 12 months post-treatment.

The second study (Koushik et al., 2009) provided the LP to 12 children between the ages of 6 years 8 months and 10 years 8 months (mean 9 years 0 months) at the start of treatment.

Pre-treatment, audio-recorded speech samples of spontaneous conversation with the clinician were obtained for each child in the clinic 1–2 weeks prior to the start of treatment. Children were excluded if the %SS was less than 2.0 at the pre-treatment assessment, and English was not the most proficient language. Follow-up assessments were conducted 9–187 weeks post-treatment (mean 70 weeks). These assessments were done by telephone calls to the children at home, by a graduate student in speech pathology. Each child was telephoned three times randomly at home within a 7–10 day period. All samples were audio recorded. Each conversation was about 10 minutes long, and the child was asked open-ended questions. This method was chosen for its validity in preference to parents and children returning to the clinic for follow-up. It is well known that the latter would incur potential bias from discriminated learning to the clinic setting, and possible participant selection bias of those parents who were willing to return to the clinic (Ingham, 1981). Calls were made at random by a stranger and were chosen because of their potential for higher demand characteristics in preference to having a parent record the child's speech. Additionally, parents were interviewed about their experiences with the LP.

Pre- and post-treatment speech measures were %SS and stuttering severity. Stuttering severity was measured on a 10-point perceptual scale where 1 = no stuttering, 2 = extremely mild stuttering and 10 = extremely severe stuttering (Onslow et al., 2003). Measures were made by independent, blinded observers.

The therapy was parent administered and closely approximated standard delivery of the LP with preschool children. The criteria for ending Stage 1 of the treatment reflected the manualised LP at the time:[2] (1) %SS below 1.0 in the clinic, and (2) severity rating scores for the previous week of '1' each day for either three consecutive visits or two consecutive clinic visits spanning a 3-week period during which there was an intervening non-attendance at the clinic.

One child required a supplement to the LP. This child received the addition of a speech restructuring component in addition to the LP and his results were eliminated from the group results.

The children reduced their stuttering from a pre-treatment mean of 9.2–1.9 %SS at follow-up. Despite large stuttering reductions at follow-up, three of the children had stuttering rates that were greater than 3.0 %SS. Reliability between the blinded observers and the clinician observers was 0.91 ($p < 0.001$).

These results were obtained in a median of eight clinic visits (range 6-10). The blind observer's mean speech rate scores in SPM was 145.8 (SD 22.7) pre-treatment and 179.3 (SD 20.5) at follow-up. This result is consistent with improved verbal output associated with stuttering reduction and also indicates that stuttering reductions were not attained at the cost of reduced speaking rate. No association was found between follow-up period and stuttering rates, suggesting the durability of treatment effects. Figure 5.1 provides the individual data for 11 children comparing pre-treatment to follow-up %SS.

Parents in both Koushik et al. (2009) and Lincoln et al. (1996) reported being satisfied with their children's post-treatment speech. Koushik et al., interviewed parents of ten of the children about their satisfaction with the LP. Using the 10-point severity scale, seven parents assigned a score of 1 or 2 to their child's speech at follow-up, indicating no or extremely mild stuttering. Three parents assigned scores of severity 3. Eight parents reported that their child's stuttering had not worsened since the last clinic visit and two reported a slight increase. Eight parents said they continued to provide occasional verbal contingencies for both stutter-free and stuttered speech. Although all parents enjoyed participating in the LP, six also said that they found it difficult to find time to conduct treatment during structured conversations because of busy home schedules.

It is somewhat difficult to compare the results of Koushik et al. (2009) to that of Lincoln et al. (1996), which was based upon an earlier version of the LP

---

[2]See footnote on p. 58. The current Packman et al. (2011) treatment guide excludes measures of %SS as a criterion for Stage 2 entry and progression.

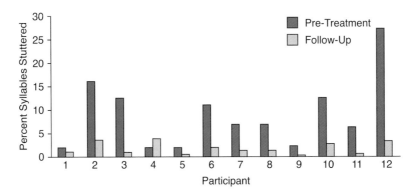

Figure 5.1 Pre-treatment and follow-up percent syllables stuttered scores for the 12 children in the Koushik et al. (2009) report. Note that Child 11 entered Stage 2 with more liberal criteria than specified with the trial protocol. Child 12 required a speech restructuring treatment adjunct (Koushik et al., 2009).

with this age group. While the possibility of a large effect size was reported for both studies, more replication is certainly needed. Koushik et al.'s study may contain positive bias in participant selection because of its retrospective nature. Another limitation is the comparison of in-clinic recordings in the pre-treatment assessment with telephone recordings at the post-treatment follow-up. Although seven children did not achieve the LP criteria at the time for preschool children of %SS less than 1.0 at follow-up, reductions in stuttering were significant for the majority.

The results of a recent case study of an Iranian school-age boy who received the LP (Bakhtiar and Packman 2009) were consistent with the two studies reviewed previously. %SS during the first clinic visit were presented graphically with the boy's clinic chart, and were around 12 at the first clinic visit. Subsequent improvements began during subsequent, consecutive clinic visits, with reductions to 10, 8 and 5 %SS. At the conclusion of Stage 1, two independent observers measured his stuttering rate to be below 1.0 %SS during recorded conversations beyond the clinic.

In spite of the limitations of these preliminary studies, these findings pertain to an age group less likely than a preschool-age group to experience natural recovery (Yairi and Ambrose, 2005) that eliminates a source of bias.

Advantages and disadvantages

Given that stuttering becomes less tractable after the preschool years, it is clear that an efficacious stuttering treatment for school-age children is of great importance. Verbal response contingent procedures such as the LP are not complicated by programmed instruction, the use of reduced speaking rate or a novel speech pattern. The spontaneous increase of speech rate post-treatment found by Koushik et al. (2009) verifies that claim, and implies that a simple treatment for school-age children is feasible.

The findings of preliminary studies with school-age children justify the need for further clinical trials to establish treatment effects of the LP for this age group. It has been shown that procedurally, a simple treatment like the LP is viable for school-age children and that parents report enjoyment in administering the treatment. In all but one of the 12 children studied, it required no modification to the manualised procedures for school-age children and treatment time to Stage 2 was not longer than that reported for preschool-age children. These results substantiate the Lincoln et al.'s (1996) findings of an earlier version of the LP with this age group and support continued exploration of the LP with young school-age children in subsequent clinical trials.

Although four of the 11 participants maintained an average %SS below 1% at follow-up, seven others did not achieve this criterion, suggesting that there is more variability in Stage 2 outcomes for the school-age population compared to preschool children (Jones et al., 2005). This stuttering severity is comparable with the findings obtained for school-age children from Lincoln et al. (1996) study. The findings of the Lincoln et al. (1996) and Koushik et al. (2009) studies combined suggest that the LP with school-age children may not produce stuttering reductions that are as low as those seen in preschool-age children. This raises questions about what factors might contribute to this poorer outcome in the school-age population. There may be a need to adjust the criteria for entering Stage 2 for this age group, to reflect the potential inability of some school-age children with chronic persistent stuttering to reach the criteria of no stuttering. Since stuttering that persists becomes more resistant to treatment and more complex in nature, some school-age children may be unable to meet the criteria established for the preschool-age group.

While the results of Koushik et al. (2009) are encouraging, the study was preliminary and retrospective, and therefore, likely to contain positive bias associated with behaviours sought by the researchers, by self-selection of speech sampling situations. One limitation of the study is that the pre-treatment and post-treatment measures were not comparable due to the retrospective nature of the study. Additionally, non-speech data would enhance future studies as other variables related to stress and anxiety may affect stuttering in this age group.

One of the encouraging findings for the children in the Koushik et al. (2009) and Lincoln et al. (1996) studies is the number of treatment sessions required. The treatment time of a median eight clinic visits was shorter than those required for preschool-age children, which is around 11 clinic visits to Stage 2. Some explanations for this includes enhanced cognitive function in older children. This may lead to increased capacity for self-monitoring/self-correction, which is not an expectation for the preschool-age children, and may account for a faster treatment time.

Additionally, the ability of the child to participate more actively in the clinical process, through activities that include self-monitoring or self-rating of severity, may have accounted for treatment gains noted even though the children were away from their parents for large parts of the day.

If future studies find this to be an efficacious treatment it would be a welcome addition to the repertoire of the school-age clinician. Benefits of this programme in a school setting would include the short treatment time, and the lack of attention to a novel speaking condition.

Conclusions and future directions

It is worth pursuing the LP with school-age children. Hopefully further studies will continue to provide important information about the characteristics of treatments that are effective and efficacious for this age group. Conducting a prospective replication with a second school-age group would be a positive initial step. This could be followed by a Phase II clinical trial that would serve as a follow-up to the Lincoln et al. (1996) study.

Since persistent stuttering is often characterised by changes in attitudes that may influence treatment outcome, it would be worthwhile evaluating those non-speech improvements that may occur as a result of this treatment. Future studies could include evaluation of attitudes and social anxiety.

It is interesting to speculate about the predictors of best child fit to this approach, and if individual differences such as other speech and language concerns, attention deficit or other co-morbid factors affect treatment outcome. Future research might establish whether such variables are associated with improved clinical compliance and involvement of both the child and parent in a positive way.

More information regarding the use of the LP with school-age children in effectiveness of generalising fluency from within- to beyond-clinic settings is needed. Perhaps a part of that information will be whether children of this age are reliable in collecting their own stuttering severity ratings during everyday life, particularly at school.

Discussion

Ann Packman
This is a question from the sceptics in our group. Koushik et al. (2009) was not a prospective study. Might there have been other children who dropped out or for whom it wasn't successful? Were the children in that study taken from the waiting list in consecutive order?

Rosalee Shenker
It was a respective study of long-term outcomes of 12 children taken in consecutive waiting list order, and there were no dropouts.

Joseph Attanasio
How does you definition of school age as 7-12 years correspond with the Canadian school system?

Rosalee Shenker

School age for us is defined by the period, in Canada, Grade 1 to Grade 6 before secondary education starts so that would be approximately from 7 to 12 years.

Joseph Attanasio

And is there any differential responsiveness to the treatment during that period?

Rosalee Shenker

I find that the best age within that range for LP treatment is 7–9 years, but that is just my opinion without any research to back it up. I would say that the window closes around 11 years onwards, were we find at the Montreal Fluency Centre that there are better programmes to use, as children get closer to adolescence.

Sheena Reilly

We were intrigued about whether the children were formally requested to self-monitor as part of the programme and if so was that home, school or generally?

Rosalee Shenker

No, not in the Koushik et al. (2009) study. But when we looked at the results for that group of children we made some changes to the way we provide the treatment. Now our procedure is that children of that age, who receive the LP, as well as their parents, collect their own severity scores outside the clinic and bring them each week. We find that useful because, although there is general consistency between parent and child severity scores, often there would be one day where the scores would be different. The child would often experience a lot more stuttering that the parent would record. Parents would often say something like 'gosh, I didn't hear you stuttering so much that day, what happened, why did you give yourself that score?' and the child would say something like 'because I had to do a presentation in front of the class and I bombed and it was really horrible'. And the parent inevitably would say something like 'I am so glad I know that, next time I can help you with that'. Clinically, that seems to work really well.

Sheena Reilly

At what age do you think you could start that self-monitoring and self-assessment with children?

Rosalee Shenker

I think safely I could say 7 years, perhaps even a bit younger depending on the cognitive ability of the child.

Ann Packman

We were wondering whether any of the children had previously had the LP treatment and whether you think that might be a help or a hindrance if they had, and especially if they might have failed before.

Rosalee Shenker

None of them had any prior LP treatment. But I don't recall whether any of them had any other previous treatment.[3]

Joseph Attanasio

Could you tell us if you have identified any characteristics of the children that make them particularly good candidates for the LP at this age or not good candidates?

Rosalee Shenker

One thing that seems to make them good candidates is that this is the treatment that they want to do. Not when parents want the treatment and the children were unsure, but when children state their compliance. For me, that really stands out as being one important characteristic of this age group that is related to the treatment success. Also, the development of spontaneous self-monitoring.

Sheena Reilly

Do you know anything about the children's stuttering at school?

Rosalee Shenker

Not from the Koushik et al. (2009) study. But clinically, the children's severity scores that I mentioned just then, that are currently part of our clinical routine, give us that information. I find such child measures are critical because of the variability of stuttering across childhood situations.

Ann Packman

We were also interested to know if, when children 7–9 years become markedly fluent after LP treatment, they still have some lingering negative speech attitudes and situation avoidance. Also, if they had been teased and bullied, did that just stop with the arrival of stuttering reduction?

Rosalee Shenker

That is something that we didn't investigate. Of course it would have been better to but it was a retrospective study and we did not have pre-treatment measures of such things. For future studies I do think these measures need to be built in. Obviously it is most important to evaluate with this age group. I must say though that the issue never came up in the clinic with the children and very often when there is an issue the children will tell us, then we respond to it.

Joseph Attanasio

With preschool children treated with the LP, two studies indicated that the treatment does not have a frank effect on language development (Bonelli et al., 2000; Lattermann et al., 2005). In other words, the children were not sacrificing language for fluency. In the older age group where the children

---

[3]The Koushik et al. (2009) report states nothing about the treatment history of the children.

may be more sensitive to what they are doing, is there any sense that they might be sacrificing not language development but length and complexity of utterance for fluency? In other words, do you think the kids are shortening and simplifying their utterances to be more fluent?

Rosalee Shenker

I don't have any idea about that but of course we have the post-treatment samples and we could get some information from those. I do have data on a group of school-age children that we followed up 4–7 years after the LP and we analysed their conversation speech samples and their development was consistent with their age (Shenker and Roberts, 2006).[4]

Sheena Reilly

Could you talk a little bit more about the follow-up periods, which I think had quite a range, from 9 to 187 weeks with an average of 79 weeks. We were intrigued as to whether there could be a relationship between the time at which you followed up and the outcome?

Rosalee Shenker

We did that analysis and in the paper reported that there was no relation between duration of follow-up and outcome in terms of stuttering severity.

Ann Packman

You mentioned that one child received some adjunct speech restructuring component. What would be the criteria for introducing that? How long would you wait? The Koushik et al. (2009) paper reported such a strategy for only one child of the 12. Would you anticipate that clinicians would encounter more children than that needing such a strategy?

Rosalee Shenker

The reason this child received the speech prolongation addition was that the parent requested it after becoming a little unmotivated and non-compliant with the LP. At the Montreal Fluency Centre we have a chart review of every child who is receiving the LP, regardless of age, at about 5 weeks after the treatment starts. If we are not getting a treatment effect then we do some troubleshooting to try and understand why. For preschool children that almost invariably fixes the problem. For school-age children, if that does not fix the problem, we do another chart review at about 11 or 12 weeks and if the child is still not making progress with the standard LP, then we will consider changing the nature of the therapy. This is a new policy for us.

Joseph Attanasio

You said that treatment time was shorter for these school-age children than preschoolers who typically receive LP treatment. Apart from rate of progress, are there any other differences in treatment responsiveness?

---

[4]Onslow et al. (2001) also reported linguistic data for two school-age boys whose stuttering was controlled with time-out during a previous laboratory study. During time out conditions, one boy reduced his language complexity and one did not.

Rosalee Shenker

What comes to mind is that I would say with the older children they more quickly get down to a severity rating of around 3–4 and we will often see progress stalled at that point. I don't know why, but that is often the time when we have to do a chart review to find out what is causing it. Sometimes the child just becomes unmotivated by the verbal contingencies and we have to explore a change in the verbal contingencies. Sometimes the parent is not using the verbal contingencies much because the child is stuttering less. Sometimes we can fix this with a tangible reward system. Often we can fix it by simply increasing the number of verbal contingencies that the child receives.

Sheena Reilly

You highlighted that one of the problems with the Koushik et al. (2009) data was the different methods for collecting the pre-treatment and post-treatment measures. Would you design the study differently if you were doing it again prospectively? Could you comment on whether you think this design flaw had any impact on how you interpret the outcomes from the study?

Rosalee Shenker

I guess we don't know. But what I can say is that we had a rigorous post-treatment assessment by telephone that would have revealed all the post-treatment stuttering that was present.

Ann Packman

What are your future research plans? Where are you going from here with the LP for this age group?

Rosalee Shenker

I'm in the same position as those at the Institute for Stuttering Treatment and Research (see Chapter 9). The Montreal Fluency Centre is a specialist treatment unit with very little research funding. What research we can do is thanks to the generosity of the clinicians that work with me and spend their time willingly evaluating these programmes. That aside, I think that one of the things that I would like to do is a prospective study of the LP with school-age children but with a more comprehensive set of measures, particularly including non-speech measures. I would also like to trial the LP against one of the more traditional therapies. I am also interested in the language abilities of these older children and how that might affect treatment outcomes, along with cognitive capacity.

Joseph Attanasio

Do you have any idea why that one child worsened after treatment?

Rosalee Shenker

Yes, it was parent compliance. The parent stopped providing the verbal contingencies during Stage 2. Commonly, that may cause stuttering to increase and that is what happened on this occasion.

Joseph Attanasio

Is it true that child finished up with more severe stuttering than before treatment?

Rosalee Shenker

Yes, that is the case, but I am not sure it could be attributed to the LP.

Sheena Reilly

Given that the LP has been around for quite some time, our group were intrigued with why it has not been trialled much with school-age children. Is it just simply that it's promoted as a programme for young children and nobody has been adventurous enough to do it with school-age children?

Rosalee Shenker

I haven't really thought about it. In my experience many clinicians are happy to try it with that age group, but I have certainly heard little about plans by researchers for prospective clinical trials.

Ann Packman

We were wondering about what effect the positive attention to speech might have. Could that be part of the treatment effect, possibly a major part?

Rosalee Shenker

It is true that the LP causes parents to spend more quality time with their children with all kinds of novel activities. Parents tell us that it encourages them to enjoy their children, and the children certainly benefit from this different kind of attention. But to what extent that is a treatment effect is an empirical question. I don't think it is possible to know any other way but with experimentation.

References

Andrews, G., Guitar, B., & Howie, P. (1980) Meta-analysis of the effects of stuttering treatment. *Journal of Speech and Hearing Disorders, 45,* 287–307.

Bakhtiar, M., & Packman, A. (2009) Intervention with the Lidcombe Program for a bilingual school-age child who stutters in Iran. *Folia Phoniatrica et Logopaedica, 61*(5), 300–304.

Block, S., Onslow, M., Roberts, S., & White, R. (2004) Control of stuttering with EMG feedback. *Advances in Speech Pathology, 6,* 100–106.

Bloodstein, O., & Bernstein Ratner, N. (2008) *A Handbook on Stuttering* (6th ed.). Clifton Park, NY: Delmar.

Boberg, E., & Kully, D. (1994) Long-term results of an intensive treatment program for adults and adolescents who stutter. *Journal of Speech and Hearing Research, 37,* 1050–1059.

Bonelli, P., Dixon, M., Bernstein Ratner, N., & Onslow, M. (2000) Child and parent speech and language following the Lidcombe Program of early stuttering intervention. *Clinical Linguistics and Phonetics, 14,* 427–446.

Bothe, A. K. (2004) *Evidence-Based Treatment of Stuttering: Empirical Bases and Clinical Applications.* Mahwah, NJ: Lawrence Erlbaum Associates.

Bothe, A. K., Davidow, J. H., Bramlett, R. E., & Ingham, R. J. (2006) Stuttering treatment research 1970–2005. I. Systematic review incorporating trial quality assessment of behavioral, cognitive, and related approaches. *American Journal of Speech-Language Pathology, 15*, 342–352.

Bridgman, K., Onslow, M., O'Brian, S., Block, S., & Jones, M. (2011) Changes to stuttering measurement during the Lidcombe Program treatment process. *Asia Pacific Journal of Speech, Language, and Hearing, 14,* 147–152.

Budd, K. S., Madison, L. S., Itzkowitz, J. S., George, C. H., & Price, H. A. (1986) Parents and therapists as allies in behavioral treatment of children's stuttering. *Behavior Therapy, 17*(5), 538–553.

Craig, A., Hancock, K., Chang, E., McCready, C., Shepley, A., McCaul, A. (1996) A controlled clinical trial for stuttering in persons aged 9 to 14 years. *Journal of Speech and Hearing Research, 39*, 808–826.

de Kindkelder, M., & Boelens, H. (1998) Habit-reversal treatment for children's stuttering: assessment in three settings. *Journal of Behavioral Therapy and Experimental Psychiatry, 29*(3), 261–265.

Hancock, K., Craig, A., McCready, C., McCaul, A., Costello, D., Campbell, K., & Campbell, K. (1998) Two- to six-year controlled-trial stuttering outcomes for children and adolescents. *Journal of Speech Language and Hearing Research, 41*(6), 1242–1252.

Harrison, E., & Onslow, M. (2009) The Lidcombe Program for preschool children who stutter. In: B. Guitar & R. McCauley (Eds.), *Treatment of Stuttering: Established and Emerging Interventions* (pp. 118–140). Baltimore, MD: Lippincott Williams and Wilkins.

Howie, P. M., Tanner, S., & Andrews, G. (1981) Short-term and long-term outcome in an intensive treatment program for adult stutterers. *Journal of Speech and Hearing Disorders, 46*, 104–109.

Huber, A., O'Brian, S., Onslow, M., & Packman, A. (2003) Results of a pilot study of EMG biofeedback for the control of stuttering in adolescents. Proceedings of the 2003 Speech Pathology Australia Conference, Hobart, Australia; pp. 177–182.

Ingham, R.J. (1981) Evaluation and maintenance in stuttering treatment: a search for ecstasy with nothing but agony. In: E. Boberg (Ed.), *Maintenance of Fluency* (pp. 179–218). New York: Elsevier.

Ingham, R. J., & Cordes, A. K. (1999) On watching a discipline shoot itself in the foot: some observations on current trends in stuttering treatment research. In: N. B. Ratner & C. E. Healey (Eds.), *Stuttering Research and Practice: Bridging the Gap* (pp. 211–230). Mahwah, NJ: Lawrence Erlbaum Associates.

Jones, M., Onslow, M., Packman, A., Williams, S., Ormond, T., Schwartz, T., & Gebski, V. (2005) Randomized controlled trial of the Lidcombe Program of early stuttering intervention. *British Medical Journal, 331*, 659–661.

Koushik, S., Shenker, R., & Onslow, M. (2009) Follow-up of 6–10 year old children after Lidcombe Program treatment: a Phase I trial. *Journal of Fluency Disorders, 34*, 279–290.

Lattermann, C., Shenker, R. C., & Thordardottir, E. (2005) Progression of language complexity during treatment with the Lidcombe Program for early stuttering intervention. *American Journal of Speech-Language Pathology, 14*, 242–253.

Lincoln, M., Onslow, M., Lewis, C., & Wilson, L. (1996) A clinical trial of an operant treatment for school-age children who stutter. *American Journal of Speech-Language Pathology, 5*, 73–85.

Martin, R. (1981) Introduction and perspective: review of published research. In: E. Boberg (Ed.), *Maintenance of Fluency: Proceedings of the Banff Conference* (pp. 1–30). New York: Elsevier.

Martin, R., & Berndt, L. A. (1970) The effects of time-out on stuttering in a 12 year old boy. *Exceptional Children, 37,* 303-304.

Martin, R. R., Kuhl, P., & Haroldson, S. (1972) An experimental treatment with two preschool stuttering children. *Journal of Speech and Hearing Research, 25,* 743-752.

Onslow, M. (1996) *Behavioral Management of Stuttering.* San Diego, CA: Singular Publishing Group.

Onslow, M., Costa, L., Andrews, C., Harrison, E., & Packman, A. (1996) Speech outcomes of a prolonged-speech treatment for stuttering. *Journal of Speech and Hearing Research, 39,* 734-749.

Onslow, M., Harrison, E., & Packman, A. (2003) *The Lidcombe Program of Early Stuttering Intervention: A Clinician's Guide.* Austin, TX: Pro-Ed.

Onslow, M., & Packman, A. (Eds.) (1999) *The Handbook of Early Stuttering Intervention: A Clinician's Guide.* Austin, TX: Pro-Ed.

Onslow, M., Packman, A., Stocker, S., van Doorn, J., & Siegel, G. M. (1997) Control of children's stuttering with response contingent time-out: behavioral, perceptual and acoustic data. *Journal of Speech, Language and Hearing Research, 40,* 121-133.

Onslow, M., Ratner, N., & Packman, A. (2001) Changes in linguistic variables during operant, laboratory control of stuttering in children. *Clinical Linguistics and Phonetics, 15,* 651-662.

Packman, A., & Attanasio, J. S. (2004) *Theoretical Issues in Stuttering.* New York: Psychological Press.

Packman, A., Onslow, M., Webber, M., Harrison, E., Lees, S., Bridgman, K., & Carey, B. (2011) The Lidcombe Program of early stuttering intervention treatment guide. Retrieved from http://sydney.edu.au/health_sciences/asrc/health_professionals/asrc_download.shtml

Perkins, W. (1981) Implications of scientific research for the treatment of stuttering: a lecture. *Journal of Fluency Disorders, 6,* 155-162.

Prins, D., & Ingham, R. J. (1983) *Treatment of Stuttering in Early Childhood: Methods and Issues.* San Diego, CA: College-Hill Press.

Reed, C. G., & Godden, A. L. (1977) An experimental treatment using verbal punishment with two preschool stutterers. *Journal of Fluency Disorders, 2,* 225-233.

Ryan, B. P. & Van Kirk Ryan, B. (1983) Programmed stuttering therapy for children: comparison of four establishment programs. *Journal of Fluency Disorders, 8,* 291-321.

Ryan B. P., & Van Kirk Ryan, B. (1995) Programmed stuttering treatment for children: comparison of two establishment programs through transfer, maintenance and follow-up. *Journal of Speech and Hearing Research, 38,* 61-75.

Shenker, R. C. & Roberts, P. (2006) Long-term outcome of the Lidcombe Program in bilingual children. Proceedings of the International Fluency Association 5th World Congress on Fluency Disorders.

Wohlert, A. B., & Smith, A. (2002) Developmental change in variability of lip muscle activity in speech. *Journal of Speech, Language and Hearing Research, 45,* 1077-1087.

Yairi, E., & Ambrose, N. (2005) *Early Childhood Stuttering.* Austin, TX: Pro-Ed.

Chapter 6

Intensive Speech Restructuring Treatment for School-Age Children

Elizabeth A. Cardell
University of Queensland, Brisbane, Australia

Overview

Managing the 7–12-year-old school-age child who stutters represents a challenge for clinicians and researchers. Although the last two decades has seen much attention directed towards developing and investigating treatments for the preschool child and adults, the research into treatment effectiveness for the school-age child remains relatively scant, being often anecdotal (Guitar and McCauley, 2010) and limited to a small cohort of empirically sound studies (Nippold, 2011).

From a developmental perspective, the school-age child is unique. Indeed, why straightforward operant treatments such as the Lidcombe Program (Bakhtiar and Packman, 2009; Koushik et al., 2009; Lincoln et al., 1996) work well for some children who stutter aged 7–12 years, whilst speech restructuring (see Preface for a definition of this term) treatments seem to be required for others (Boberg and Kully, 1994; Craig et al., 1996), probably relates to aspects of maturational development that are yet to be fully elaborated. Therefore, a clinician may choose to use either a simple or complex treatment, depending on the client. However, here the focus is on speech restructuring and specifically intensive treatment formats with children. Arguably, intensive speech restructuring might be considered useful if a child has a poor response to operant treatment techniques, has moderate to severe stuttering or is in the older range of the school years.

Historically, variants of speech restructuring treatments, named variously as prolonged speech (Ingham, 1984), smooth speech (Craig et al., 1987) and precision fluency shaping (Webster, 1980), broadly evolved from the ameliorative effects of legato speech on stuttering (Wingate, 1975), which employs a

---

The Science and Practice of Stuttering Treatment: A Symposium, First Edition. Edited by Suzana Jelčić Jakšić and Mark Onslow.

slow rate, and stretching out of words that occurred during Goldiamond's (1965) seminal research about delayed auditory feedback (DAF). Indeed, speech restructuring treatments have the strongest evidence base for adults who stutter (Andrews et al., 1983; Bernstein-Ratner, 2010; Bothe et al., 2006; Onslow et al., 2008). An intensive service delivery model has been implemented in many speech restructuring programmes worldwide, with the duration ranging from 1 week (e.g. Block et al., 2005; Craig et al., 1996) to 3 weeks (e.g. Boberg and Kully, 1994; Ingham and Andrews, 1973), with Harrison et al. (1998) using one 12-hour day. Some programmes have incorporated a residential component (e.g. Ingham and Andrews, 1973; Onslow et al., 1996).

During speech restructuring treatment, clients learn to modify some or all of the parameters of breathing, phonation, articulation and prosody in order to promote continuous speech flow and airflow, and eliminate muscle tension. To learn the new techniques, speech restructuring generally incorporates programmed instruction, but this is not always the case, with an exception being the Camperdown Program (see chapter Chapter 2) (Carey et al., 2010; O'Brian et al., 2003). However, there have been no reports of the Camperdown programme being used with school-age children, so the operational characteristics of this programme will not be elaborated further. Reports of the following speech restructuring programmes have included school-age children: Boberg and Kully (1994); Budd et al. (1986); Craig et al. (1996); Druce et al. (1997); Onslow et al. (1996)[1].

Instatement

Different kinds of programmed instruction are used in different programmes. The child's new speech targets might relate to breathing, gentle onsets to phrases, light contacts of articulators, continuous airflow, continuous speech flow, continuous vocalisation, vowel lengthening, phrasing, prosody and rate control. The pertinent features of the new speech pattern are often then embedded into progressive practice at the sound, word, phrase and sentence levels, with repetition, reading and responsive naming, moving towards monologue and conversation tasks. Generally, there are criteria pertaining to either the time or number of trials under which stutter-free speech must be achieved before progressing to the next level. Slow speech rates of around 40-50 syllables per minute (SPM) are often used at the outset, with rate increasing incrementally to normal-sounding levels over the course of about 3 days with a 5-day programme, or 1 week for a 2-3-week programme. Notably, Druce et al. (1997) used clinician modelling rather than explicit teaching of targets to instate the speech technique with their 6-8-year-old children, and started this teaching at 100-120 SPM.

Attention to natural-sounding speech is a key element in most intensive speech restructuring programmes for children (Craig, 2010). If individuals do not like how they sound or perceive their speech as being unnatural, they

---

[1]The Onslow et al. report included two school-age children but it is not possible to identify their data in the report.

will be less inclined to use their fluency techniques (Menzies et al., 2009). In some programmes, naturalness is targeted as speech rates become faster (Druce et al., 1997; Onslow et al., 1996) while in others, naturalness and typical-sounding prosody is trained from the outset (Craig et al., 1996). Central to most programmes are self-evaluation activities that facilitate the child's development of self-monitoring and self-management skills. In addition to speech restructuring, anxiolytic procedures have been embedded into some programmes, with some specific cognitive restructuring tasks being built into the Craig et al. (1996) and Boberg and Kully (1994) treatments. Craig et al. also incorporated relaxation training.

Some speech restructuring intensive programmes for children conduct the majority of instatement in groups (e.g. Boberg and Kully, 1994; Craig et al., 1996), while other programmes incorporate individual therapy along with group work (Budd et al., 1986; Druce et al., 1997; Onslow et al., 1996). The Craig et al. (1996) intensive programme was largely group based. However, before attending the programme, all children received approximately 5 hours of pre-intensive individual treatment in which the smooth speech fundamentals were trained.

Transfer

Transfer of the new fluent speech pattern occurs from the first day in many programmes through home-based evening tasks. However, once the child's new fluency skills are stable at more normal-sounding speech rates, more formal transfer activities begin, using a graded exposure approach according to their individual speech situation hierarchies. The children monitor their speech during transfer tasks, using audio recordings, self-reflections and ratings.

Post-intensive maintenance

Maintenance is an essential element of the continuum of care when using intensive speech restructuring. For example, in Craig et al.'s (1996) programme, 4-hour long group maintenance sessions occurred monthly for the first 3 months post-treatment, then every 3 months up until 12 months. The sessions were formatted as 'mini-intensives', and the children brought audio-taped assignments and self-evaluations to the clinic. Budd et al. (1986) used a more home-based maintenance protocol, followed by 1-day follow-ups at 2 and 6 months post-treatment. Both Onslow et al. (1996) and Druce et al. (1997) used performance-contingent schedules with increasing time between clinic visits when programme targets were maintained.

Theoretical basis

Symptom reduction formed part of the early rationale behind using speech restructuring techniques with adults (Andrews et al., 1980; Goldiamond, 1965). Brain imaging research has demonstrated that induced fluency conditions, such as chorus reading, ameliorate stuttering by acting to attenuate the abnormal over-activations and under-activations that occur in the cerebrum and cerebellum during the stuttering moment (Braun et al., 1997; Fox et al., 1996). More recently, brain activation changes following intensive fluency-shaping therapies for adults have been demonstrated (e.g. De Nil, 1999; De Nil et al., 2003; Neumann et al., 2003, 2005) and have shown increased activations post-treatment in left hemisphere speech-relevant areas in the vicinity of pre-treatment functional deficits, and/or re-lateralisation and reductions in hypothetically compensatory right hemisphere activations.

Arguably, then, speech restructuring treatment can be said to be supported by evidence that (1) the stuttering moment represents temporal destabilisation of the neural processes that underpin planning, initiating, sequencing, executing or monitoring of speech units and movements (also see Watkins et al., 2008), and that (2) this destabilisation can be controlled, to a large extent, at a proximal level by adjusting various speech parameters.

From a neurobiological perspective, we know that in the domain of speech-language development, the synaptic overgrowth and associated superplasticity that peaks in the young brain, reduces markedly by around 7 years of age as language networks are stabilised and myelinated, and unused connections are eliminated or 'pruned' (Couperus and Nelson, 2006; Weyandt, 2006). Notably, experience determines which connections will be strengthened and which ones will be pruned. In fact, from around age 5 years, much of synaptic pruning occurs across the brain and then levels off at puberty, by which time about 40% of brain synapses have been eliminated (Chechik et al., 1998). Further, it is between the ages of 5 and 11 that the greatest increases in cortical thickness occur in the perisylvian regions (Sowell et al., 2004). Given the rapidly changing brain from early childhood to adolescence, it is possible that response to fluency treatment might vary in line with developmental aspects. In considering the time-course of some basic mechanisms of maturation and learning, intensive speech restructuring treatments appear to fit in with some of the pertinent neurobiological factors for children aged 7–12 years.

A further aspect relates to the intensive nature of the treatment and its theoretical links to motor learning and neuroplasticity. Learning is the process of neural self-modification and altered brain connections in response to experience. For connections to be strengthened, they must be used (Kolb, 1995; Maas et al., 2008). Speech restructuring is essentially motor speech learning and the re-parameterisation of motor schema (Schmidt, 1975) in generalised motor plans that are disrupted. The intensive therapy format can enhance acquisition and retention of motor skills through the neuroplasticity principles of use it to improve it, use it or lose it, repetition and specificity (Kleim and Jones, 2008; Ludlow et al., 2008; Maas et al., 2008). Importantly, for the school-age child, where synaptic pruning is a dominant process (Chechik et al., 1998), and perisylvian networks are being established and consolidated, intensive practice of fluent speech and non-practice of stuttering would appear to be important.

Table 6.1 Overview of speech restructuring reports that have included school-age children.

	Participant numbers	Age range in years	Duration
Craig et al. (1996)	Unknown[a]	Unknown[a]	1 week
Craig et al. (1996)	Unknown[a]	Unknown[a]	1[b] day a week for 4 weeks
Boberg and Kully (1994)	6	11–12	3 weeks
Budd et al. (1986)	12	7–12	1 week
Druce et al. (1997)	15	7–8	5 days

[a]The report specifies only means and age ranges, hence, it is not possible to know how many children were in the age range 7–12 years.
[b]This trial had two arms, this one involving parents attending the clinic 1 day per week.

Intensive treatment may be important, too, in light of some recent neuroimaging evidence from Chang et al. (2008) that has shown that 9–12-year-old children who stutter do not show the right hemisphere anatomical and functional increases in speech-related homologues that adults who stutter exhibit. This finding raises the possibility that the right hemisphere anomalies represent compensatory mechanisms. Under this proposition, perhaps there is a window of opportunity for the school-age child to develop fluency before stuttering becomes permanently entrenched and compensation arises. Perhaps intensive treatment might provide a requisite expediency. As things currently stand from a clinical viewpoint, using speech restructuring with a child implies an assumption or clinical judgement that stuttered speech has become, or is becoming, neurally entrenched (Craig, 2010; Guitar, 2006) and has become a skill deficit. However, this may not be the entire picture.

Demonstrated value

Despite the fact that children were not the original target group for most of the early speech restructuring research, some promising outcomes for school-age children with intensive treatment formats have emerged in five clinical reports (Boberg and Kully, 1994; Budd et al., 1986; Craig et al., 1996; Druce et al., 1997; Onslow et al., 1996). These reports are overviewed in Table 6.1. They are all non-randomised designs, and only in the case of the Druce et al. (1997) report did the report deal exclusively with children in the 7–12-years age range.[2] All treatment formats were intensive. Two of them used additives to the speech restructuring treatment: Budd et al. (1986) used DAF (see Chapter 3) and Druce et al. used a gradual increase in length and complexity of utterance (GILCU) (see Chapter 17).

[2]One was almost 7 years, at 6 years 9 months.

As shown in Table 6.1, there have been five reports of the efficacy of intensive speech restructuring with school-age children. Thus far, the most promising evidence for the efficacy of intensive speech restructuring with children has come from Craig et al.'s (1996) Phase II non-randomised controlled clinical trial. In this trial, participants were assigned to one of either a standard or parent-focused speech restructuring programme or a no-treatment control group (an EMG biofeedback group was also used but is not discussed here). Both speech restructuring treatment formats provided positive and similar stuttering reductions.

These outcomes are shown in Figure 6.1. A limitation of Figure 6.1 is that it contains data for children 7-14 years old, and may not be representative of the school-age group 7-12 years. However, assuming that it is representative, immediately post-treatment the children showed significant reductions in stuttering, with a mean percent improvement in fluency of 95% across conversation, telephone and home measures. Percent improvement reduced to 72% at 1 year post-treatment, with approximately one-third stuttering in the range of 5-18 percent syllables stuttered (%SS), indicating significant relapse (Hancock and Craig, 1998). Nonetheless, measures of speech naturalness and state and trait anxiety improved post-treatment and those gains were reasonably well maintained at 1 year post-treatment. At 5 years follow-up, percent improvement was 76% and parent reports indicated that approximately one-third of children had shown no relapse (Hancock et al., 1998). However, around 13% of children had relapsed back to pre-treatment levels of stuttering (Craig, 2010).

Boberg and Kully (1994) reported marked reductions in stuttering for the six 11-12-year-old participants in their study, which also included adolescents and adults undergoing the same treatment. Prior to treatment, the mean stuttering levels for the six children were 12.9 %SS, which reduced to 1.2 %SS

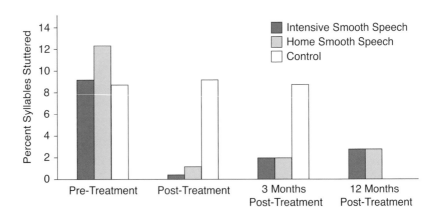

Figure 6.1 %SS for children in the Craig et al. (1996) trial treated with speech restructuring, and corresponding scores for a control group. Adapted by permission of the American Speech-Language-Hearing Association.

immediately post-treatment. At 4 months post-treatment, levels remained low at 1.8 %SS, and at 1 year post-treatment, the mean level was 2.8 %SS.

Budd et al.'s (1986) intensive programme, which incorporated DAF to train the new speech pattern, also demonstrated positive treatment effects for all the children in the study, some of which were school age. Again assuming these trends represent those for the school-age participants, the pre-treatment stuttering mean was 9.0 percent of total words spoken when talking to parents, reducing to 5.0 percent immediately post-treatment and 5.9 percent at 6 months post-treatment. Druce et al. (1997) reported a marked mean drop of stuttering to 1.8 %SS immediately post-treatment, rising 3.8 %SS at 18 months post-treatment (data specifically for two school-age children).

Advantages and disadvantages

Advantages

Intensive speech restructuring treatment has some advantages. The intensive training model ensures constant and intentional use of the speech restructuring techniques to promote acquisition of improved fluency, and constant and repetitive practice in theory facilitates change in neural circuitry (Maas et al., 2008). Many clinicians report that it is highly motivating for children and parents to see the rapid change in fluency that intensive programmes usually bring, and this gives them a sense of control and hope.

Intensive speech restructuring programmes can be convenient for children, especially when conducted in a blocked week in school holiday times. Indeed, attrition rates reported in the studies reviewed have been low. Therapy within a group context is a further strength. For the school-age child, group learning is cognitively, behaviourally, socially and educationally salient and promotes naturalistic communication opportunities. Importantly, the group setting can offer a powerful support network and, as such, can facilitate vicarious motor and cognitive learning, as well as desensitisation and disclosure, self-awareness and emotional resilience. Indeed, the emotional support that the group setting offers is valuable at this age, when stuttering-related fears, anxieties and avoidances may have emerged (Guitar, 2006; Murphy et al., 2007).

Disadvantages

However, there are a number of potential shortcomings with using intensive speech restructuring with the school-age child. Our lack of knowledge about what represents the optimal method of intensive speech restructuring means that some programmes (Boberg and Kully, 1994; Craig et al., 1996) generically modify many parameters of the speech process; however, not all children might need all parameters to achieve fluency. Indeed, in Druce's et al. (1997), therapy was delivered with clinician models with no explicit targets being taught, but it must be remembered that this programme was for younger

6-8-year-old children and the results many not necessarily be generalisable to older children.

The permanency of and neural change and automaticity of the new techniques following a 1-week or 3-week programme has to be questioned, because relapse rates for children following a 1-week programmes can be quite high, as previously discussed (see Craig et al., 1996; Hancock et al., 1998). Possibly, based on the results of (Boberg and Kully, 1994), this may be less of a problem following a 3-week programme.

Another issue is that the cognitive load to learn the complex multi-component processes of restructured speech is very high, as is the demand to summon newly instated fluency techniques in everyday situations. As such, the programmes necessitate high levels of concentration, motivation and commitment in an age group where attentional control and some aspects of insight are not yet fully developed (Weyandt, 2006).

A further barrier is that if a child's post-treatment speech sounds unnatural, or they perceive it to be unnatural, they will be less likely to use their fluency enhancing speech pattern. Unfortunately, despite the best endeavours with naturalness training and rating scales (Ingham and Onslow, 1985), there is no evidence that children feel that speech with high levels of naturalness does not feel 'different' to them.

Intensive speech restructuring programmes for children require clinicians with quite specialised expertise, as well as organisational systems and service providers that support intensive treatment models. Currently, in Australia, there are limited public resources for such programmes in education and child health settings. Added to this, some people might argue that the large number of clinical hours per child is neither time nor cost effective.

From a research perspective, it has been 15 years since the publication of Craig et al.'s (1996) study, and yet there has been no replication of this study for school-age children, either with randomised or non-randomised methods. Gaining a clear understanding of speech restructuring effectiveness with the school-age child has been difficult by the inclusion of unidentified children older than 12 years in studies.

Conclusions and future directions

There is evidence to suggest that intensive speech restructuring programmes have merit for school-age children who stutter. However, stronger and clearer evidence is needed through well-controlled studies that specifically target the 7-12-year-old age group. In addition to addressing issues of how best to facilitate acceptance of a new speech pattern and how best to prevent and manage relapse, further research is required to determine guidelines for using speech restructuring rather than simple operant methods with this age group.

In addition, further exploration is required into the issue of treatment dosage and how intensive does speech-restructuring treatment need to be for children. For example, Craig et al.'s (1996) study involved a semi-intensive

arm, and yielded comparable, if not superior, outcomes to the fully intensive programme. Also, we need to understand more about how explicit the
restructured treatment targets need to be and how best to teach these. Interestingly, similar to the Camperdown Program, the Druce et al. (1997) treatment
entailed no explicit training of multi-component speech targets. Further, it is
not clear whether all children need to be taught all parameters of the speech
restructuring technique during treatment. Finally, as the difficulties with using brain imaging with children begin to be resolved, research here would
be helpful to increase our understanding of how intensive speech restructuring, and other treatments, affect the child's brain and its structure and function. This could lead to new therapy perspectives and refinements of existing
treatments.

Discussion

Ann Packman

One of the pressing things that came up during our discussion was the treatment process. How do you instate the speech pattern, how do you shape,
generalise and maintain it? Is a treatment manual available so the current
Mater Hospital and University of Queensland[3] treatment could be replicated
in clinical practice and clinical trials?

Libby Cardell

The manual for the treatment is available and can be purchased from the Mater
Hospital in Brisbane.[4] Instatement with the speech pattern occurs individually
so when children enter the Intensive Phase they can speak stutter-free at
50 SPM or less. I am currently in the process of developing a slightly different
manual as well. Our manual continually evolves.

Sheena Reilly

The first thing we would like to ask you about is parent involvement. In the
Craig et al. (1996) trial you mentioned two speech-restructuring arms: a 5-day
intensive, and a 1 day per week treatment involving parents. We were intrigued
that the parent-based programme is not the treatment that you presently give
at the University of Queensland, since it had equivalent, if not better, outcomes
to the 5-day intensive.

Libby Cardell

Instead of a fully home-based programme, what we do at present is to get the
parents more involved than occurs with the more traditional types of speech
restructuring programmes. We train the parents as well as the children to

---

[3]Associate Professor Cardell currently conducts the treatment at, and in conjunction
with, the University of Queensland. She will be conducting this treatment through Griffith
University, as well.
[4]Readers wishing to do so can contact Associate Professor Cardell at
e.cardell@griffith.edu.au.

do the speech pattern and they are required to practice regularly with their children. Some kind of home component is essential for speech restructuring treatment to work with school-age children.

Joseph Attanasio

You raised the theoretical prospect that the reported success of this treatment with some children is connected with synaptic pruning. We would like to know how you might test any hypotheses that might derive from that position.

Libby Cardell

I am thinking it through now, actually. The manual that I mentioned that I am currently developing is based on motor learning principles.

Joseph Attanasio

But that is programme development. I meant are you planning any research, or can you suggest any research, that would confirm or refute the underlying causes you propose for the effects of this treatment with school-age children.

Libby Cardell

I am thinking a lot about that. I am interested in looking at stuttering during this age range in terms of speech motor development. With a child who is 7 or 8, one assumes that they have developed general motor plans for speech, but there are these little parameters of force, timing and space, perhaps, that are dissociable from that that are somehow being disrupted. I am interested in exploring force, timing and space; those dissociable parameters of generalised motor plans. I am not sure yet how that exploration will occur. I am currently discussing the matter with a colleague at the University of Queensland. Perhaps those who stutter do not always do the same stutter. It may well be that for some, the parameter of force is more of an issue. Perhaps there is a timing versus a space issue. Of course, these are only speech motor concerns. Other points of vulnerability, which I am researching, deal with lexical access using event-related potential. So I am trying to understand the underpinnings at multiple levels. I am just identifying my research areas at present, but am excited about all that potential.

Ann Packman

We were interested that you have such an intensive stage of treatment and whether that is actually necessary. And we were also interested to know how you endeavour to ensure that children continue, during their everyday lives, to use the speech pattern they have learned.

Libby Cardell

Obviously, it comes down much to individual choice with how much children use the speech technique, how much they feel they need to use it and how much they are prepared to use it. But the whole issue of intensity fascinates me, and I am really keen to explore differences between a multiday intensive and an intensive 12-hour day. We need to optimise the acquisition of clinical skills and the use of clinical resources. Additionally, there are models of human learning that would suggest the need for a period to consolidate. Perhaps it would be better to have 2 days, then a break to allow for memory consolidation and whatever, and then maybe another couple of days. Clearly, internalisation for internal control is an important facet of encouraging acquisition and retention in learning. Currently I am discussing this issue with another colleague at the University of Queensland, not just in relation to stuttering, but for dysarthria and apraxia as well.

Ann Packman

Do you have a systematic maintenance programme with regular visits, and do you measure or assess the children's use of the requisite speech pattern during that period?

Libby Cardell

Yes, definitely. Children and parents can attend for weekly individual sessions or group sessions. With the individual maintenance sessions, they have to bring in recorded evidence of their use of the speech pattern and self-ratings of their stuttering severity in various situations.

Ann Packman

How long is the maintenance programme?

Libby Cardell

We don't do the performance-contingent type of maintenance that others do. Essentially, as long as the child and parent need external support, we have a policy that 'the door is never closed'.

Sheena Reilly

I want to go back to the theory issue again. We talked a lot about this and what you described as theory of the treatment mechanism. We wanted to ask you this. Given the rates of relapse of this population in clinical trials – similar to that occurring for adults – could you not simply be teaching compensation methods rather producing motor re-learning?

Libby Cardell

I think that is a fair comment. I described imaging changes in the brains of people who stutter. In one of those studies (Neumann et al., 2005) there was increased left-sided activity immediately after the intensive programme. So is that the effects of compensation or motor learning? The right hemisphere has been found to be more under-activated after these sorts of therapies (Neumann et al., 2003) and so it may be not so much compensation but more motor learning. I think evidence from brain imaging supports that to an extent.

Joseph Attanasio

What is the aim of the programme? Is it to have children become fluent to the point where they don't depend on a speech technique? Or is it that they must remain somewhat vigilant in order to not stutter?

Libby Cardell

It would be wonderful if there were some way that we could use therapy with this age group while their brains are still plastic so that the amount of attention and vigilance that they have to put into speech, ultimately, is diminished to extremely low levels. Once you get to adulthood or adolescence, really that vigilance never seems to leave the person who stutters. I don't know the answer to this, so what I will say is that if there is a way, and if it is related to treatment intensity and neurobiology, I think, at least, we have to start to think about that. Being able to rewire the brain in a positive way at a younger age will mean less of that vigilance later during life. That whole area needs research.

Ann Packman

Our group was interested to find out what you think are the active components of the treatment, because there seem to be many components.

Libby Cardell

I think that obviously the slowed rate is a key factor. I believe that what we call 'chunking' is a big factor too because that allows children to plan what to say next and to keep their thoughts a lot more organised, and possibly to settle the brain back to a resting level before speaking again. 'Blending', as we call it, is very important but probably one of its most important aspects are gentle onsets and easing into phrases.

Ann Packman

And how do you think the anxiolytic component of the treatment contributes?

Libby Cardell

This is of course a critical research area. For now, however, I have an intuitive clinical belief that the anxiolytic procedures and cognitive restructuring contributes to anxiety reduction and avoidance reduction. But the contribution of these features to documented treatment effects in children is yet to be known.

Sheena Reilly

Can all 7–12-year olds cope with 5 days of 8-hour treatment per day?

Libby Cardell

It does require a certain degree of readiness and aptitude from the children and there are some for whom this treatment is not appropriate.

Sheena Reilly

So who are the children for whom you would not recommend it? That is the critical issue.

Libby Cardell

Children who have significant language or speech problems as well as stuttering. Also, children who have hyperactivity deficits. But not necessarily children who are slower to learn because what we have found is that the initial learning of the speech technique can occur individually in our programmes so they can have the time to take longer to learn. We have flexibility with the programme as well where the children with other issues might attend for perhaps 3 days for shorter hours with fewer demands in terms of the transfer tasks and possibly more time spent on the actual instatement. We don't want to exclude any child.

References

Andrews, G., Guitar, B., & Howie, P. (1980) Meta-analysis of the effects of stuttering treatment. *Journal of Speech and Hearing Disorders, 45,* 287-307.

Andrews, G., Craig, A., Feyer, A.-M., Hoddinot, S., Howie, P., & Neilson, M. (1983) Stuttering: a review of research findings and theories circa 1982. *Journal of Speech and Hearing Disorders, 48,* 226-246.

Bakhtiar, M., & Packman, A. (2009) Intervention with the Lidcombe Program for a bilingual school-age child who stutters in Iran. *Folia Phoniatrica et Logopaedica, 61,* 300-304.

Bernstein-Ratner, N. (2010) Translating recent research into meaningful clinical practice. *Seminars in Speech and Language, 31,* 236-249.

Block, S., Onslow, M., Packman, A., Gray, B., & Dacakis, G. (2005) Treatment of chronic stuttering: outcomes from a student training clinic. *International Journal of Language and Communication Disorders, 40,* 455-466.

Boberg, E., & Kully, D. (1994) Long-term results of an intensive program for adults and adolescents who stutter. *Journal of Speech and Hearing Research, 37,* 1050-1059.

Bothe, A. K., Davidow, J. H., Bramlett, R. E., & Ingham R. J. (2006) Stuttering treatment research 1970-2005: I. Systematic review incorporating trial quality assessment of behavioral, cognitive, and related approaches. *American Journal of Speech-Language Pathology, 15,* 321-341.

Braun, A. R., Varga, M., Stager, S., Schultz, G., Selbie, S., Maisog, J. M., & Ludlow, C. L. (1997) Altered patterns of cerebral activity during speech and language production in developmental stuttering. An H2(15)O positron emission tomography study. *Brain, 120,* 761-784.

Budd, K. S., Madison, L. S., Itzkowitz, J. S., George, C. H., & Price, H. A. (1986) Parents and therapists as allies in behavioural treatment of children's stuttering. *Behaviour Therapy, 17,* 538-553.

Carey, B., O'Brian, S., Onslow, M., Block, S., Packman, A., & Jones, M. (2010) Randomised controlled non-inferiority trial of a telehealth treatment for chronic stuttering: the Camperdown Program. *International Journal of Language and Communication Disorders, 45,* 108-120.

Chang, S. E., Erickson, K. I., Ambrose, N. G., Hasegawa-Johnson, M. A., & Ludlow, C. L. (2008) Brain anatomy differences in childhood stuttering. *Neuroimage, 39,* 1333-1344.

Chechik, C., Meliljson, I., & Ruppin, E. (1998) Synaptic pruning in development: a computational account. *Neural Computation, 10,* 1759-1777.

Couperus, J. W., & Nelson, C. A. (2006) Early brain development and plasticity. In: K. McCartney & D. Phillips (Eds.), *Blackwell Handbook of Early Childhood Development* (pp. 85-105). Malden, MA: Blackwell Publishing.

Craig, A. (2010) Smooth speech and cognitive behavioural therapy. In: B. Guitar & R. McCauley (Eds.), *Treatment of Stuttering: Established and Emerging Interventions* (pp. 188-214). Baltimore, MD: Lippincott Williams and Wilkins.

Craig, A., Feyer, A. M., & Andrews, G. (1987) An overview of a behavioral treatment for stuttering. *Australian Psychologist, 22,* 53-62.

Craig, A., Hancock, K., Chang, E., McCready, C., Shepley, A., McCaul, A., & Reilly, K. (1996) A controlled clinical trial for stuttering persons aged 9 to 14 years. *Journal of Speech and Hearing Research, 39*, 808-826.

De Nil, L. F. (1999) Stuttering: a neurophysiological perspective. In: N. Bernstein-Ratner & C. Healey (Eds.), *Stuttering Research and Practice: Bridging the Gap* (pp. 85-102). Mahwah, NJ: Erlbaum.

De Nil, L. F., Kroll, R. M., Lafaille, S. J., & Houle, S. (2003) A positron emission study of short- and long-term treatment effects on functional brain activation in adults who stutter. *Journal of Fluency Disorders, 28*, 357-380.

Druce, T., Debney, S., & Byrt, T. (1997) Evaluation of an intensive treatment program for stuttering in young children. *Journal of Fluency Disorders, 22*, 169-186.

Fox, P. T., Ingham, R. J., Ingham, J. C., Hirsch, T. B., Downs, J. H., Martin, C., & Lancaster, J. L. (1996) A PET study of the neural systems of stuttering. *Nature, 382*, 158-162.

Goldiamond, I. (1965) Stuttering and fluency as manipulatable operant treatment classes. In: L. Krasner & L. Ullmann (Eds.), *Research in Behavior Modification* (pp. 106-156). New York: Holt, Reinhart and Winston.

Guitar, B. (2006) *Stuttering: An Integrated Approach to its Nature and Treatment* (3rd ed.). Baltimore, MD: Lippincott Williams and Wilkins.

Guitar, B., & McCauley, R. (2010) *Treatment of Stuttering: Established and Emerging Interventions*. Baltimore, MD: Lippincott Williams and Wilkins.

Hancock, K., & Craig, A. (1998) Predictors of stuttering relapse one year following treatment for children aged 9 to 14 years. *Journal of Fluency Disorders, 23*, 31-48.

Hancock, K., Craig, A., Campbell, K., Costello, D., Gilmore, G., McCaul, A., & McCready, C. (1998) Two to six year controlled trial stuttering outcomes for children and adolescents. *Journal of Speech and Hearing Research, 41*, 1242-1252.

Harrison, E., Onslow, M., Andrews, G., Packman, A., & Webber, M. (1998) Control of stuttering with prolonged speech: development of a one-day instatement program. In: A. Cordes and R. Ingham (Eds.), *Treatment Efficacy in Stuttering* (pp. 191-212). San Diego, CA: Singular Publishing Group.

Ingham, R. J. (1984) *Stuttering and Behavior Therapy*. San Diego, CA: College Hill.

Ingham, R. J., & Andrews, G. (1973) Details of a token economy stuttering therapy for adults. *Australian Journal of Human Communication Disorders, 1*, 13-20.

Ingham, R. J., & Onslow, M. (1985) Measurement and modification of speech naturalness during stuttering therapy. *Journal of Speech and Hearing Disorders, 50*, 261-281.

Kleim, J. A., & Jones, T. A. (2008) Principles of experience-dependent neural plasticity: Implications for rehabilitation after brain damage. *Journal of Speech, Language, and Hearing Research, 51*, S225-S239.

Kolb, B. (1995) *Brain Plasticity and Behavior*. Mahwah, NJ: Erlbaum.

Koushik, S., Shenker, R., & Onslow, M. (2009) Follow-up of 6-10-year old stuttering children after Lidcombe Program treatment: a Phase 1 trial. *Journal of Fluency Disorders, 34*, 279-290.

Lincoln, M., Onslow, M., Lewis, C., & Wilson, L. (1996) A clinical trial of an operant treatment for school-age children who stutter. *American Journal of Speech-Language Pathology, 5*, 73-85.

Ludlow, C. L., Hoit, J., Kent, R., Ramig, L. O., Shrivastav, R., Strand, E., & Sapienza, C. M. (2008) Translating principles of neuroplasticity on speech motor control and recovery. *Journal of Speech, Language, and Hearing Research, 51*, S240-S258.

Maas, E., Robin, D. A., Austerman Hula, S. N., Freedma, S. K., Wulf, G., Ballard, K. J., & Schmidt, R. A. (2008) Principles of motor learning in treatment of motor speech disorders. *American Journal of Speech-Language Pathology, 17,* 277-298.

Menzies, R., Onslow, M., Packman, A., & O'Brian, S. (2009) Cognitive behavior therapy for adults who stutter: a tutorial for speech-language pathologists. *Journal of Fluency Disorders, 34,* 187-200.

Murphy, W. P., Yaruss, J. S., & Quesal, R. W. (2007) Enhancing treatment for school-age children who stutter I. Reducing negative reactions through desensitization and cognitive restructuring. *Journal of Fluency Disorders, 32,* 121-138.

Neumann, K., Euler, H. A., Wolff von Gudenberg, A., Giraud, A. L., Lanfermann, H., Gall, V., & Prebisch, C. (2003) The nature and treatment of stuttering as revealed by fMRI: A within- and between group comparison. *Journal of Fluency Disorders, 28,* 381-410.

Neumann, K., Prebisch, C., Euler, H. A., Wolff von Gudenberg, A., Lanfermann, H., Gall, V., & Giraud, A. L. (2005) Cortical plasticity associated with stuttering therapy. *Journal of Fluency Disorders, 30,* 23-39.

Nippold, M. A. (2011) Stuttering in school-age children: a call for treatment research. *Language, Speech, and Hearing Services in Schools, 42,* 99-101.

O'Brian, S., Onslow, M., Cream, A., & Packman, A. (2003) Camperdown Program: outcomes of a new prolonged speech treatment model. *Journal of Speech, Language and Hearing Research, 46,* 933-946.

Onslow, M., Costa, L., Andrews, C., & Harrison, E. (1996) Speech outcomes of a prolonged speech treatment for stuttering. *Journal of Speech and Hearing Research, 39,* 734-739.

Onslow, M., Jones, M., O'Brian, S., Menzies, R., & Packman, A. (2008) Defining, identifying, and evaluating clinical trials of stuttering treatments: a tutorial for clinicians. *American Journal of Speech-Language Pathology, 17,* 401-415.

Schmidt, R. A. (1975) A schema theory of discrete motor skill learning. *Psychological Review, 82,* 225-260.

Sowell, E. R., Thompson, P. M., Leonard, C. M., Welcome, S. E., Kan, E., & Toga, A. W. (2004) Longitudinal mapping of cortical thickness and brain growth in normal children. *Journal of Neuroscience, 24,* 8223-8231.

Watkins, K. E., Smith, S. M., Davis, S., & Howell, P. (2008) Structural and functional abnormalities of the motor system in developmental stuttering. *Brain, 131,* 50-59.

Webster, R. L. (1980) Evolution of a target-based behavioral therapy for stuttering. *Journal of Fluency Disorders, 5,* 303-320.

Weyandt, L. N. (2006) *The Physiological Bases for Cognitive and Behavioural Disorders.* Mahwah, NJ: Lawrence Erlbaum Associates, Inc.

Wingate, M. E. (1975) *Stuttering: Theory and Treatment.* New York: Irvington.

Chapter 7

Student-Delivered Treatment for Stuttering: Multiday Intensive Speech Restructuring

Susan Block
La Trobe University, Melbourne, Australia

Overview

Graduates from speech pathology programmes are the lifeblood of our profession. Emerging evidence suggests that we may have underestimated the prevalence of stuttering with recent estimate of a cumulative incidence of 8.5% in 3-year-old children (Reilly et al., 2009). Consequently, it is vital that graduates from speech pathology courses are well prepared to work with people of all ages who stutter. There is evidence that new graduates will choose to work with client groups with whom they feel confident and to whom they have had clinical exposure during their professional preparation programmes (St. Louis and Durrenberger, 1993). What follows is an outline of an integrated academic, clinical and research programme to prepare undergraduate and postgraduate speech pathology students to work with people of all ages who stutter.

The School of Human Communication Sciences at La Trobe University in Melbourne, Australia offers undergraduate and postgraduate speech pathology programmes. Clinical experience of stuttering for both groups of students occurs during their final year. The School provides a community clinic, which aims to offer evidence-based best practice, supervised student-delivered treatment for people of all ages who stutter. Under supervision, students present the Lidcombe Program (Packman et al., 2011) to preschool children. School-age children receive the Lidcombe Program and other treatments. Adolescents and adults receive an intensive speech-restructuring (see Preface for a definition of this term) programme (Block et al., 2005). Students have

The Science and Practice of Stuttering Treatment: A Symposium, First Edition. Edited by Suzana Jelčić Jakšić and Mark Onslow.

also recently presented an alternative speech restructuring programme, which is an adaptation of the Camperdown Program (CP; O'Brian et al., 2001, 2003) designed to meet the restrictions of a 10-week student clinical placement.

Prior to participating in the clinic, students have received approximately 50 hours of academic classes related to stuttering theory, assessment and treatment. They have also attended a clinical observation of an assessment or treatment of someone who stutters, completed speech measurement training and visited a meeting of a self-help group for people who stutter.

The clinical experience described in the following text is the intensive Smooth Speech Program. Smooth Speech is a method of speech restructuring. It is a 'speak-more-fluently' approach (Boberg, 1981) whereby the individual who stutters is taught a different way of speaking, which is incompatible with stuttering. Clients learn to prevent stuttering from occurring by restructuring their speech production. Smooth Speech is a variant of prolonged speech (Ingham, 1984). It is commonly used for adolescents and adults who stutter (Andrews et al., 1983; Block et al., 2005; Boberg and Kully, 1994).

Description of programme

The La Trobe Intensive Smooth Speech Program is a 2-month programme. The initial component is a 5-day intensive course conducted by supervised final year student clinicians, who attend from 8.30 am to 7.00 pm daily. Most of the treatment during this initial phase is individual with group practice opportunities occurring generally twice each day. The programme incorporates the routine speech restructuring strategies of gentle onsets, elongating vowels and joining words together. Participants commence with fluent production of isolated consonants and vowels and then various vowel–consonant combinations before they attempt connected speech using the requisite speech pattern. Once they begin connected speech they progress through speaking tasks at gradually increasing faster rates, increasing usually from 60 syllables per minute to approximately 200 syllables per minute. There is a focus on speech naturalness throughout all the tasks, particularly when speech rate increases to normal levels. The intensive programme is followed by seven consecutive weekly 2-hour sessions. These include 1.5 hours of individual treatment and a 1/2 hour of group fluency practice.

The programme incorporates fluency instatement followed by transfer and generalisation activities for 1 or 2 days. This is followed by seven weekly maintenance sessions. Each programme involves 12–16 participants with 24–32 student clinicians and three or four supervising clinicians. The programmes are offered to adolescents and adults but the age groups are not combined for any one programme.

Following the programme, participants are encouraged to attend a review day twice a year. More than 50% choose to attend in the year following their intensive programme. This review day also is student delivered. The review days incorporate approximately 6 hours of individual treatment aimed at reviewing fluency strategies and problem-solving strategies to enhance generalisation and maintenance.

Students are required to plan and report on each session they conduct. They have an assessment of their clinical performance at mid-placement. At the end of the placement there is a final collaborative assessment in which they are required to meet the predetermined professional competency level of 'independence' (Speech Pathology Australia, 2001).

Theoretical basis

Student education

St. Louis and Durrenberger (1993) reported findings that a lack of education and insufficient clinical experience were the reasons most commonly given for why specific disorders are those least preferred by speech pathology clinicians in America. Those clinicians who listed stuttering as one of their most preferred disorders were more likely to have had experience during their student years working with people who stutter than those clinicians who listed stuttering as least preferred. Similarly, Kelly et al. (1997) described insufficient clinical education and minimal coursework as reasons for clinician apprehension towards stuttering. More recently, Yaruss and Quesal (2002) found results consistent with an earlier study (Yaruss, 1999), that many graduate students do not receive sufficient education in the area of fluency disorders. They reported that almost two-thirds of the staff from programmes stated that it is possible for students to graduate without any clinical experience in stuttering. In Australia, Speech Pathology Australia has included fluency as one of the five key areas in which all graduates must have direct clinical experience (Speech Pathology Australia, 2001).

Treatment

Goldiamond (1965) created a significant impact on the treatment of stuttering in adults. His work led to a renewed focus on changing how the person who stuttered spoke. Goldiamond reported on the use of delayed auditory feedback (DAF) in single-subject laboratory experiments. The resulting elongated speech pattern established the fact that DAF could control stuttered speech, and that the slow and unnatural speech pattern could be shaped to resemble normal speech. The speech pattern change treatments that were derived from the DAF investigations by Goldiamond have been know with various terms as overviewed by Ingham (1984).

At the same time as Goldiamond (1965) was experimenting with DAF, researchers such as Shames and Sherrick (1963) and Martin and Siegel (1966) were experimenting with operant conditioning. The combination of the operant methodology and stuttering control using DAF induced stuttering control led to international treatments incorporating both approaches (Ingham, 1984).

That development influences treatments of today, with intensive speech restructuring conducted by many centres (Andrews et al., 1980; Block et al., 2005; Boberg and Kully, 1994).

Demonstrated value

Intensive Smooth Speech Programs during the past two decades at The School of Human Communication Sciences at La Trobe University have contributed participants to clinical trials. This has the educational advantage that students are learning to simultaneously incorporate research protocols into their routine clinical practice. The first was a trial of the student education clinic against international clinical trial benchmarks (Block et al., 2005). Subsequent trials reported the benefits of adding two components to the standard protocol: cognitive behaviour therapy (Menzies et al., 2008) and self-modelling (Cream et al., 2010).

The Block et al. (2005) clinical trial is the best evidence for the efficacy of the La Trobe student-delivered treatment model. Participants were 78 adults who stutter, of whom 66 were men and 12 were women. The mean age was 28 years and the age range was 18-70 years. Speech assessments were conducted 1 week and 1 day before the start of the treatment programme. Post-treatment assessments were conducted immediately following the intensive component of the programme, then 3 months, 12 months and then 3.5-5 years post-treatment.

For assessments up to 12 months post-treatment, participants provided 10-minute beyond-clinic audio-taped speech samples. These were people known to them, telephone calls from their homes and conversations in their homes. During the period 3.5-5 years post-treatment, an investigator telephoned the participants unexpectedly and audio recorded a 10-minute conversation. Recordings were also made in the clinic during the period of the study. Results at all assessments showed that stuttering rates in the clinic were around twice those recorded at home. For the home recordings, pre-treatment stuttering rates were in the range of 2-4 percent syllables stuttered (%SS), and were well below 2.0 %SS at 12 months post-treatment and 1.6 %SS at 3.5-5 years post-treatment. Speech naturalness data from stutter-free speech segments were obtained immediately post-treatment, and suggested some compromise in order to control stuttering, but not excessively so compared to other reports. In short, results were equivalent to benchmark data from other clinical trials of intensive speech restructuring treatment. Results are presented in Figure 7.1.

To demonstrate the adaptability of a student education clinical model, a modification of the Camperdown Program (O'Brian et al., 2003) (see Chapter 2) was designed to fit into that model at La Trobe (Cocomazzo et al., 2011). The adapted model involved 26 weeks of treatment during 10 weeks by 24 student clinicians. There were two, 2-hour individual teaching sessions followed by one

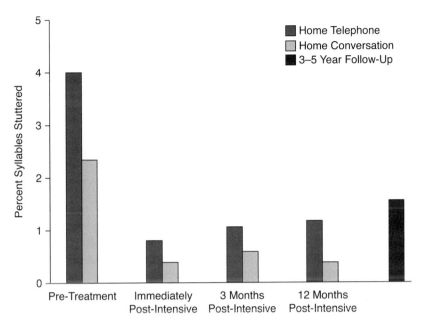

Figure 7.1 Mean pre-treatment and post-treatment assessment results from the Block et al. (2005) trial. Assessments up to 12 months post-treatment are percent syllables stuttered (%SS) from two beyond-clinic recordings. %SS scores at 3.5–5 years post-treatment are based on one unexpected telephone call to participants (Block et al., 2005).

8-hour group practice day. This was followed by seven 2-hour problem-solving sessions. Twelve adults undertook the programme: 10 men and two women, with a mean age of 29 years and a range of 21–47 years. Outcomes were reported pre-treatment, immediately post-treatment and 12 months post-treatment by means of within-clinic recordings with a clinician and beyond-clinic recordings with familiar people. Again, the La Trobe student education model produced benchmark outcomes. %SS beyond the clinic was 5.5 pre-treatment and 1.2 and 2.1 immediately post-treatment and 12 months post-treatment, respectively. Speech naturalness analyses provided essentially similar results to Block et al. (2005).

Advantages and disadvantages

Advantages

A significant advantage of speech restructuring treatments such as those outlined previously is that people who stutter can quickly learn strategies to speak fluently. Importantly, large numbers of clients can be treated simultaneously. They experience massed practice opportunities to change their speech motor pattern. While participating in intensive treatment when others with the same problem attend at the same time, there are frequent opportunities to meet and practise with others struggling with the same issues: they experience support and camaraderie from others in the group. This can provide opportunities for education, support and desensitisation. Intensive treatment allows for much change during a short period. This in itself can be strongly motivating for an individual who has grappled with stuttering over many years.

From an academic and clinical perspective, students experience all aspects of the treatment process. They experience both assessment and all stages of the treatment process: fluency instatement, transfer, maintenance and the virtually inevitable need to deal with relapse. One of the most important advantages of these clinical placement experiences is that students have access to supervisors who are specialists in stuttering treatment. Indeed, participants in the Block et al. (2005) and Cocomazzo et al. (2011) trials reported enjoyment working with enthusiastic, well-prepared and well-trained students and knowledgeable clinical supervisors.

Disadvantages

Of course, rapid change from intensive speech restructuring can bring disappointment in the common event of relapse. Thus, it is important that on-going maintenance opportunities are available. This is particularly the case considering that one report has identified the presence of mental health disorders – most of which involve anxiety – determiners of whether a client will be in the two-thirds of cohorts who typically experience problems with fluency maintenance (Iverach et al., 2009). Clearly then, for some, speech restructuring alone may not be sufficient to overcome the sense of handicap that can ensue from a lifetime of stuttering (Bloodstein, 1995). As a consequence, additional and different treatment such as adjunct treatment with cognitive behaviour therapy may be appropriate (e.g. see Menzies et al., 2008).

Providing students with adequate clinical experience with stuttering is expensive and time-consuming. Clinic experiences such as those outlined previously require dedicated and experienced clinical supervisors. The need for on-going feedback, report reading and marking are onerous for the staff involved. There is a large workload for clinical supervisors. Sufficient and flexible space is required to accommodate a service delivery model such as La Trobe, where there might be up to 16 clients, 32 students and four supervisors present simultaneously. The clinic sessions are long, the work is repetitive and the supervision is expensive. In spite of these issues the learning experiences for the students are sufficiently valuable that they report them to be an enjoyable experience leading to confidence working with people who stutter.

Some challenges with student-delivered treatment for stuttering relate to limited and potentially decreasing funding, increasing student numbers, increasing demand for clinical services and pressure from university administrators to divert staff time from clinical supervision to research activity.

However, as shown with the reports outlined here, integrating research and clinical experience is one means of achieving that goal.

Conclusions and future directions

The clinical services outlined previously demonstrate that large numbers of students, well supervised, can provide an effective clinical service for large numbers of adolescents and adults who stutter. They can achieve positive speech outcomes for their clients. They can impact their client's well-being and quality of life. A flexible and varied service delivery has provided a range of valuable experiences for both clients and students. Students embrace these experiences enthusiastically. Based at least on the reports reviewed here, it is evident that people who stutter will come to university clinics for treatment. Because research is a significant part of university life, clients are usually very happy to participate in a variety of research programmes. Such programmes can be integrated into a student-delivered clinical service with impressive speech outcomes. They also provide valuable experiences for students to enhance what they will do when they enter the workforce following graduation. They also provide valuable clinical experiences that may help students feel positive and confident about treating people who stutter.

The future challenge here is to encourage researchers to be involved in student education so that students can contribute to meaningful clinical research about the evidence-based treatments they will use during their careers. To ensure this, sufficient funding needs to be provided to ensure the careful integration of research, clinical service delivery and adequate clinical supervision. Researchers in such settings can motivate students with their expert research knowledge and clinical experience. We plan to continue a close association with researchers to collaborate on alternative treatments and service delivery options. Additionally, we are investigating ways of increasing student numbers in each clinical placement, to ensure that clinical supervisors are not overburdened and clients experience adequate continuity of care.

There is a need to make treatments for adults more accessible and as simple as possible. With regards to the former, telehealth service delivery of speech restructuring treatment is an option that is becoming more readily available and more comprehensively researched (see Chapter 10). A recent randomised controlled trial (Carey et al., 2010), conducted at the La Trobe clinic, showed this service delivery model to be equivalent to in-clinic treatment in terms of outcome. Consequently, we are incorporating telephone and webcam sessions where clients are unable to attend all sessions in the clinic. This should ensure more flexible treatment options for people who find it difficult to access treatment or to access on-going treatment. We anticipate involvement in future clinical trials of this method. With regards to treatment simplicity, the CP was developed in part to address that issue, and we anticipate participation in further clinical trials to supplement the Cocomazzo et al. (2011) report described previously.

Discussion

Joseph Attanasio

You generated many questions in our group about student training, which is something that involves many of us. Could you talk about how the students who do the therapy are trained? How they are selected and how they are supervised?

Susan Block

I present their stuttering management course during their third year, so I know exactly what they have been taught. The course is approximately 50 hours of class time. We have people who stutter coming in to talk to the students about their experience of stuttering and their experience of treatment. As part of their course they are required to go to a self-help group meeting without me or any other staff member being present, so they can discover first hand what those who stutter say about their experiences and the treatment they have received. Part of their assessment during their course is real time measurement of %SS, which is a core clinical skill for the treatments described. Their training occurs with a computer-based speech-rating package (Block and Dacakis, 2002). Additionally, they are familiar with self-rating scales such as those used with the CP. They have a 1-hour group meeting with their supervisors before the intensive programme. During that meeting they are given an outline of the programme and details of what they will be expected to do, and they have to prepare some resources. For example, the programme begins with a list of isolated consonants and vowels, and then various vowel-consonant combinations for clients to practise with the requisite speech pattern before they attempt connected speech. They prepare those lists themselves and the intention there is to have them start thinking about the processes of the programme. Then on each morning of the programme we meet with them for about 1 hour of briefing before the clients arrive. For that meeting we expect them to bring ideas and resources with them. So, for adolescents they might need to bring games and literature and things that might interest an adolescent. Supervisors, of course, watch the students working and give them real time guidance, but also students receive written feedback each day. It is critical for the students to model the speech pattern correctly for the clients, so supervisors are particularly vigilant to ensure that they do that correctly.

Ann Packman

Could you comment on something we discussed? If this symposium is any kind of guide, there are an extraordinary number of different treatments available. So you are in a no-win situation as a clinical educator. You can expose students to a range of treatments, with clinical mastery of none or have students attain professional entry-level competence in one treatment only. It just does not seem feasible for students to attain competence in more than one stuttering treatment, considering all the other speech and language disorders they have to treat. You clearly have gone down the path of seeking student clinical competence in one adult treatment only.

Susan Block

Of course during my coursework students are introduced to a wide range of treatments. But I could defend our training in one specific treatment style for students on the grounds that speech restructuring and its variants has by far the best clinical trials evidence to support it than any other adult treatment.

Sheena Reilly

You strike us as a master clinician and educator. There is no doubt what happens at your university clinic is remarkable. But we wondered whether it could be replicated. Could any of us do what you have done, or is it your charisma and strong professional motivation that is the key to your success.

Susan Block

It's a really important point because Bloodstein's (1995) well-known criteria for evaluating treatment include that the treatment has to be shown to be effective in the hands of essentially any qualified clinician. And of course students are not qualified clinicians, and I think it is important that our students can achieve results as favourable as any reported in the clinical trials literature. But to answer your question directly, the programme has been replicated as a student training clinic at the University of Sydney and at the University of Queensland.

Joseph Attanasio

You described two student clinicians per client. Could you tells us why and what the impact might be on the clients and the clinicians, and if the student clinicians give feedback to each other?

Susan Block

We do it in pairs to deal with the student numbers. A benefit of working with student pairs is that they can learn from each other. However, I constantly make the point that two student clinicians do not equal one qualified clinician. Of course, it would be much easier to work with one student per client, but that would halve the numbers of students to whom we could provide clinical education, and cause us not to meet our target of proper clinical education for them. I should say that from the client point of view, working with a pair is of students is sometimes much better than working with one, and sometimes it's the other way around. Students vary of course with skill level, so during the programme we rotate them among the clients.

Ann Packman

Just to clarify, are you saying that every La Trobe speech pathology student obtains experience in your intensive group programme?

Susan Block

No, they did once but no longer, which is something I have never become com-fortable with. All our masters students do the programme and probably about

60% of the undergraduates.[1] The majority of the undergraduates who don't do a clinical placement with the intensive programme do one with the Lidcombe Program. However, every student who requests a stuttering placement will get one, even if we need to take extra clients to manage the numbers. If they do not have a requested stuttering placement at La Trobe, we subsequently attempt to obtain one for them at some other time during their course, in a community clinic.

Sheena Reilly

We had a discussion about how the skill of an individual clinician can mediate an outcome for a client. How do you ensure quality control with your programme, given that, as you said, that not all students have equal skills?

Susan Block

A colleague who is very experienced and works in the clinic with us all the time occasionally will say that clients get better despite the students because the treatment is so powerful. But quality control is of course an issue. We have audio-visual recording facilities in the clinic, and if a student needs some feedback about clinical errors with clients we often record and play back the errors and discuss them. At the end of each lunch break, we meet with the students and go over the strengths and weaknesses with what we have seen them doing. Many of those interactions involve discussions about common student errors with counselling, such as not following through with client leads and terminating discussions prematurely.

Joseph Attanasio

You obviously have integrated research effort into your student clinical training programme. Could you divulge the secret about how you've been able to do this? It's been my experience at least that it's very difficult to convince students and their supervisors to do research. Their primary effort is to help that client and that does not leave room for much else.

Susan Block

The answer is simple. We accomplish it by means of a large group of researchers who share the load of the research, who are spread across several Australian cities. All these people contribute to the work of conceptualising, doing and writing up research. Most of the clinical trials of speech restructuring treatment in Australia have pooled participants from many clinical sites, the majority of which involve student supervision.

Ann Packman

I understand you have some anxiolytic procedures in your programme. How do the students deal with that? Is that more difficult for them to master than the speech restructuring procedures?

---

[1]At the time of the symposium, the La Trobe School of Human Sciences conducted undergraduate and postgraduate speech pathology programmes.

Susan Block

It is a little more difficult for them. A core skill for them to acquire is construction of a desensitisation hierarchy for clients, and that is far from straightforward. However, generally during the treatment anxiolytic procedures are closely linked with speech restructuring procedures so the clinical training of them is manageable during the programme. One challenge is to stop students who are interested in psychology going off on a tangent and losing the essential focus on speech restructuring. All the anxiolytic procedures we use are designed to facilitate that programme goal.

References

Andrews, G., Guitar, B., & Howie, P. (1980) Meta-analysis of the effects of stuttering treatment. *Journal of Speech and Hearing Disorders, 45,* 287–307.

Andrews, G., Craig, A., Feyer, A., Hoddinott, S., Howie, P., & Neilson, M. (1983) Stuttering: A review of research findings and theories circa 1982. *Journal of Speech and Hearing Disorders, 48,* 226–246.

Block, S., & Dacakis, G. (2002) Stuttering counts. Measuring stuttering and speech rate. Multimedia Production Unit, COMET, La Trobe University, Melbourne, Australia.

Block, S., Onslow, M., Packman, A., Gray, B., & Dacakis, G. (2005) Treatment of chronic stuttering: outcomes from a student training model. *International Journal of Language and Communication Disorders, 40,* 455–466.

Bloodstein, O. (1995) *A Handbook on Stuttering* (5th ed.). San Diego, CA: Singular Publishing Group.

Boberg, E. (1981) *Maintenance of Fluency.* New York: Elsevier.

Boberg, E., & Kully, D. (1994) Long-term results of an intensive treatment program for adults and adolescents who stutter. *Journal of Speech and Hearing Research, 37,* 1050–1059.

Carey, B., O'Brian, S., Onslow, M., Block, S., Jones, M., & Packman, A. (2010) Randomised controlled non-inferiority trial of a telehealth treatment for chronic stuttering: The Camperdown Program. *International Journal of Language and Communication Disorders, 45,* 108–120.

Cocomazzo, N., Block, S., Carey, B., O'Brian, S., Onslow, M., Packman, A., & Iverach, L. (2011) Camperdown Program for adults who stutter: A student training clinic Phase I trial. Manuscript in preparation.

Cream, A., O'Brian, S., Jones, M., Block, S. Harrison, E., Lincoln, M., et al. (2010) Randomized controlled trial of video self-modelling following speech restructuring treatment for stuttering. *Journal of Speech, Language, and Hearing Research, 53,* 1–11.

Goldiamond, I. (1965) Stuttering and fluency as manipulatable operant response classes. In: L. Krasner & L. Ullmann (Eds.), *Research in Behaviour Modification* (pp. 106–156). New York: Holt, Rinehart and Winston.

Ingham, R. J. (1984) *Stuttering and Behavior Therapy. Current Status and Experimental Foundations.* San Diego, CA: College-Hill Press.

Iverach, L., Jones, M., O'Brian, S., Block, S., Lincoln, M., Harrison, E., & Onslow, M. (2009) The relationship between mental health disorders, stuttering severity and treatment outcome among adults who stutter. *Journal of Fluency Disorders, 34,* 29–43.

Kelly, E. M., Martin, J. S., Baker, K. E., Rivera, N. I., Bishop, J. E., Kriziske, C. B., & Stealy, J. M. (1997) Academic and clinical preparation and practices of school speech-language pathologists with people who stutter. *Language, Speech and Hearing Services in Schools, 28*, 195-212.

Martin, R., & Siegel, G. (1966) The effects of simultaneously punishing stuttering and rewarding fluency. *Journal of Speech and Hearing Research, 9*, 466-475.

Menzies, R., O'Brian, S. Onslow, M., Packman, A., St Clare, T. & Block, S. (2008) An experimental clinical trial of a cognitive behavior therapy package for chronic stuttering. *Journal of Speech, Language, and Hearing Research, 51*, 1451-1464.

O'Brian, S., Cream, A., Onslow, M., & Packman, A. (2001) A replicable, non-programmed, instrument-free method for the control of stuttering with prolonged speech. *Asia Pacific Journal of Speech, Language and Hearing, 6*, 91-96.

O'Brian, S., Onslow, M., Cream, A., & Packman, A. (2003) The Camperdown Program: Outcomes of a new prolonged-speech treatment model. *Journal of Speech, Language, and Hearing Disorders, 46*, 933-946.

Packman, A., Onslow, M., Webber, M., Harrison, E., Lees, S., Bridgman, K., & Carey, B. (2011) The Lidcombe Program of Early Stuttering Intervention. Treatment Guide. Retrieved from http://sydney.edu.au/health_sciences/asrc/docs/lidcombe_program_guide_2011.pdf

Reilly, S., Onslow, M., Packman, A., Wake, M., Bavin, E. L., Prior, M., & Ukoumunne, O. (2009) Predicting stuttering onset by the age of 3 years: a prospective, community cohort study. *Pediatrics, 123*(1), 270-277.

Shames, G., & Sherrick, C. (1963) A discussion of nonfluency and stuttering as operant behavior. *Journal of Speech and Hearing Disorders, 28*, 3-18.

Speech Pathology Australia. (2001) Competency-Based Occupational Standards (CBOS) for Speech Pathologists - Entry Level. The Speech Pathology Association of Australia Limited, Melbourne. Retrieved from http://www.speechpathologyaustralia.org.au/resources/compassr

St. Louis, K. O., & Durrenberger, C. H. (1993) What communication disorders do experienced clinicians prefer to manage? *ASHA, 35*, 23-27.

Yaruss, J. S. (1999) Current status of academic and clinical education in fluency disorders at ASHA-accredited training programs. *Journal of Fluency Disorders, 24*, 169-183.

Yaruss, J. S., & Quesal, R. W. (2002) Academic and clinical education in fluency disorders: an update. *Journal of Fluency Disorders, 27*, 43-63.

Chapter 8

Review of the Successful Stuttering Management Program

Michael Blomgren
The University of Utah, Salt Lake City, UT, USA

Overview

The Successful Stuttering Management Program (SSMP) was developed in 1962 by Dorvan Breitenfeldt at Eastern Washington University (Breitenfeldt and Lorenz, 1999). The programme has been a widely recognised treatment option in United States for many years. The SSMP has its roots in the early theories and therapies of stuttering proposed by Lee Travis and Bryng Bryngelson. Later, the SSMP was influenced by the stuttering treatment approaches described by Bloodstein (1975), Johnson (1967), Sheehan (1970, 1979), Van Riper (1973) and Williams (1971). Collectively, these approaches are often referred to as *stuttering management* therapies (Blomgren, 2010). Since nearly all of these early stuttering management approaches originated at the University of Iowa, the approaches have also been termed the 'Iowa Way' (Zebrowski and Arenas, 2011). Stuttering management therapies, including the SSMP, incorporate various combinations of therapeutic techniques including *desensitisation* to stuttering and stuttering *modification* techniques to decrease the muscular tension associated with stuttering moments. An overriding goal of all stuttering management approaches is to foster acceptance of stuttering, decrease the fear and avoidance of stuttering and to stutter with less effort.

Basic elements of cognitive behaviour therapy (CBT) are also utilised in the SSMP. CBT therapy is a method of identifying and replacing fear-promoting beliefs with more rational and functional ones (see Chapter 14). The core component of CBT for people who stutter is challenging unhelpful beliefs about possible negative evaluation by listeners. CBT therapy involves systematically

The Science and Practice of Stuttering Treatment: A Symposium, First Edition. Edited by Suzana Jelčić Jakšić and Mark Onslow.

modifying negative thoughts related to stuttering and social interaction. CBT is typically used to decrease debilitating levels of social anxiety related to stuttering and speaking. Reducing anxiety is often considered an important component of stuttering treatment as approximately 50% of adults who stutter may have significantly high levels of social anxiety (Kraaimaat et al., 2002; Menzies et al., 2008). CBT may help produce less social avoidance and anxiety (Craig and Tran, 2006; Menzies et al., 2009). In this regard, stuttering management therapy like the SSMP tends to be primarily anxiolytic (anxiety reducing) in emphasis (Blomgren et al., 2005).

The SSMP is a 3-week residential programme. Group and individual therapy is offered for 3.5 hours each weekday afternoon. Clients are assigned numerous speaking tasks to complete during the mornings. Group social activities are also arranged on Saturdays. The SSMP involves approximately 65 hours of direct therapy. There are typically 6–10 clients per clinic. Over the years, the SSMP has also served as a training programme for speech-language pathology students at Eastern Washington University. Clients are assigned at least one speech-language pathology graduate student who serves as the client's primary clinician. All clients and student clinicians are typically supervised by two or more certified speech-language pathology supervisors.

The programme consists of three treatment phases: (1) confrontation of stuttering, (2) modification of stuttering and (3) maintenance. The first phase – confrontation – is the main component of treatment and lasts approximately 2 weeks. The confrontation phase is designed to modify the client's attitudes and perceptions about stuttering. Attitudes and perceptions are modified through a series of desensitisation and CBT exercises. More generally, treatment includes activities designed to help eliminate avoidance strategies. These activities include advertising one's stuttering in various speaking situations, identifying and analysing moments of stuttering and purposefully ceasing word and situation avoidance behaviours. Practice of these techniques takes place in the clinic during both group and individual treatment sessions. Practice also takes place during numerous telephone speaking tasks and extra-clinical speaking tasks such as interviewing strangers about their stuttering knowledge and beliefs.

The second phase of treatment involves learning specific techniques designed to decrease the severity of stuttering moments when they occur. These stuttering modification techniques include utterance initial phoneme prolongations, stuttering moment cancellations and 'pullouts' from stuttering moments (Breitenfeldt and Lorenz, 1999). The duration of the second phase of treatment is approximately 3 days.

The third and final phase of the SSMP is focused on establishing a maintenance plan for clients. The duration of this phase is 2 days. During this final treatment phase, clients are encouraged to continue to use their stuttering management techniques in all non-clinical speaking situations. Clients are also encouraged to maintain contact with the clinic and to join a self-help group such as a chapter of the National Stuttering Association.

Theoretical basis

As stated at the outset of this chapter, the SSMP is an example of the 'Iowa Model' of stuttering therapy. While there is very limited empirical support for Iowa-based models of therapy, the approach is grounded in a number of theoretical tenets. The primary theoretical basis for stuttering management approaches comes from two-component models of stuttering (Bloodstein and Ratner, 2008; Prins and Ingham, 2009). That is, the first component of stuttering (the overt stuttering) can lead to the second component (the affective, anxiolytic and avoidance components of stuttering). Proponents of stuttering management therapy often believe that completely decreasing overt stuttering is either very difficult or impossible. Therefore, they argue that the second component of stuttering should really be the primary objective of treatment. To a great extent the SSMP, like most desensitisation therapies, is founded in the cognitive learning literature (e.g. Bandura, 1977, 1986; Sheehan, 1951; Wolpe, 1958).

Ingham (1984) provides a good general overview of the genesis of the Iowa model. The Iowa model started in the 1930s with the work of Lee Travis and Bryng Bryngelson. Ingham states that the therapy procedures promoted by Bryngelson required both attitude change and social adjustment to enable the stutterer to cope with the assumed emotional consequences that arise from stuttering. One significant therapy procedure that Bryngelson introduced was 'voluntary stuttering'; a procedure borrowed from the Negative Practice technique introduced by Knight Dunlap (1932, p. 7).

Voluntary stuttering, or pseudo-stuttering, remains an integral component of the SSMP.

These early foundations of stuttering management therapies at the University of Iowa were further developed by Wendell Johnson and his student Dean Williams (Johnson, 1961; Williams, 1957, 1979). Johnson and Williams focused on reducing 'undesirable behaviours' that may impede fluent speech. In 1957, Dean Williams published an article called 'A Point of View about Stuttering'. This article serves as one of the earliest narratives outlining what would later come to be known as the stuttering management approach. The goal of Williams' therapy was to have the individual who stutters feel and monitor speech processes in order to improve fluency. Williams also counselled those who stutter to not view their stuttering as the thing that defines them as a person, but as merely something they do. Williams believed that when a person who stutters thinks that stuttering 'simply' happens to them, feelings of helplessness arise. The goal of this early stuttering management therapy was to teach those who stutter to modify their stuttering and to manage the disorder in positive proactive ways.

In subsequent years, Charles Van Riper (1973), another graduate of the University of Iowa, wrote about a number of additional stuttering management techniques. Van Riper advocated working on eye contact, self-disclosure of stuttering, pseudo-stuttering, freezing (holding a movement of stuttering in order to analyse it), ceasing avoidance behaviours and tolerating frustration. Most of these treatment techniques had the goal of reducing tension, anxiety and avoidance associated with stuttering. Further, Van Riper (1986) encouraged 'a bath of stuttering' in order to desensitise the stuttering speaker to their stuttering fears. The goal of stuttering desensitisation was to reduce the individual's fears of speaking and stuttering as well as to reduce frustration and shame associated with being a stutterer.

Demonstrated value

The persistent problem with stuttering management approaches such as the SSMP is that little treatment efficacy research has been conducted to show that the approach is beneficial to people who stutter (Bothe et al., 2006). Further, the limited amount of research on stuttering management techniques is relatively dated (e.g. Boudreau and Jeffrey, 1973; Dalali and Sheehan, 1974; Fishman, 1937; Gregory, 1972; Irwin, 1972; Prins, 1970). In spite of the SSMP's nearly 55-year existence, there has been little published about actual treatment outcomes. No treatment outcome data are included in the SSMP manual (Breitenfeldt and Lorenz, 1999). Two descriptive outcome studies have been published including a conference proceedings paper (Breitenfeld and Girson, 1995) and an article by Eichstadt et al. (1998). These articles described positive treatment related changes in attitudes, secondary behaviours and improvement in some speech related characteristics. However, these publications are limited by their lack of data, lack of criteria for determining significance and lack of statistical methodology. Three published reviews of the SSMP manual have outlined the structure of the programme and identified some strengths and weaknesses of the programme (see De Nil and Kroll, 1996; Ham, 1996; Manning, 1990).

Given the paucity of evidence to support the clinical effectiveness of the SSMP, a recent attempt was made to evaluate the SSMP on various treatment outcomes (Blomgren et al., 2005). Blomgren et al. (2005) independently evaluated the SSMP when it was offered at the University of Utah from 1999 to 2002. Specifically, a series of 14 fluency- and affective-based measures were used to assess the SSMP immediately after treatment and 6 months after treatment. Measures included (1) stuttering frequency, (2) the Stuttering Severity Instrument (SSI; Riley, 1994), (3) a self-rating of stuttering severity, (4) the Perceptions of Stuttering Inventory (Woolf, 1967), (5) the Locus of Control of Behaviour scale (Craig et al., 1984), (6) the Beck Depression Inventory (Beck and Steer, 1993), (7) the Multi-component Anxiety Inventory IV (Schalling et al., 1973) and (8) the State-Trait Anxiety Inventory (Spielberger et al., 1983). Results of this study indicated that the SSMP appeared to reduce a number of anxiety related features of stuttering, such as self-perceived avoidance and expectancy of stuttering, and self-reported psychic and somatic anxiety. Further, these anxiolytic reductions appeared to be durable, as measured 6 months post-treatment. However, the results also indicated

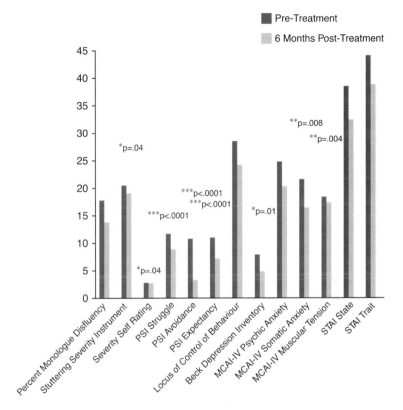

Figure 8.1 Pre-treatment and 6 month post-treatment measures for the Blomgren et al. (2005) clinical trial. Significance levels for results are based on omnibus Friedman tests for repeated observation medians during pre-treatment, immediate post-treatment and 6 months post-treatment observations. PSI, Perceptions of Stuttering Inventory; MCAI-IV, Multi-component Anxiety Inventory IV; STAI, State-Trait Anxiety Inventory. (Data from Blomgren et al. (2005).)

that no durable reductions were identified in (1) decreasing overt stuttering frequency, (2) decreasing stuttering severity (measured as a composite of stuttering frequency, stuttering moment durations and secondary behaviours (SSI-3)), (3) self-assessed stuttering severity, (4) self-assessed perception of struggle to speak, (5) self-assessed amount of muscular tension, (6) self-assessed improvement in mood, (7) self-assessed improvements in locus of control or (8) self-assessed improvements in state or trait anxiety. Based on these findings, the SSMP was deemed to be an ineffective treatment for decreasing stuttering and related muscular struggle behaviours, but it was deemed to be an effective treatment for decreasing some of the anxiolytic and avoidance aspects of stuttering. This conclusion is justified by the possibility that a non-randomised outcomes study may lead to overestimation of any effect sizes compared to the gold standard of a randomised control trial (Kunz and Oxman, 1998). Figure 8.1 summarises the results of the Blomgren et al. (2005) clinical trial.

Advantages and disadvantages

Advantages

The programme addresses the acceptance, disclosure and perception of stigma that many people who stutter find difficult. Additionally, the intensity of the treatment, the group dynamic and the 'it's OK to stutter' philosophy are positive aspects for many participants. From a historical perspective, the programme was developed with input from those who stutter. It is probably not inconsequential that Breitenfeldt is a person who stutters, as were Johnson, Van Riper and Sheehan. From an evidence-based perspective, the SSMP does appear to decrease avoidance and expectancy of stuttering as well as some forms of anxiety (Blomgren et al., 2005).

There are a number of possible weaknesses of the SSMP. The 3-week intensive nature of the treatment is cost and time prohibitive for many people who stutter. The treatment is also very dependent on the stuttering management counselling skills of the clinicians, which may influence the portability of the approach across clinicians. In this sense, the 'therapist effect' may play a larger role in stuttering management therapies than in more regimented speech restructuring approaches (Crits-Cristoph et al., 1991).

Disadvantages

The main weakness of the SSMP for many stuttering speakers may simply be that decreasing stuttering frequency is not a goal of the treatment. As such, the approach does not teach fluency-facilitating techniques and subsequently the programme does not result in decreased stuttering frequency or decreased struggle to speak (Blomgren et al., 2005). For many stuttering speakers, the singular focus on treating the anxiolytic and reactive aspects of stuttering might be viewed as insufficient – especially in light of the many available programmes that report positive results in decreasing core stuttering behaviours (Andrews et al., 1980; Blomgren, 2010; Howie et al., 1981; Ingham, 1975; Kroll and Scott-Sulsky, 2010; Kully et al., 2007; Montgomery, 2006; O'Brian et al., 2010; Ryan, 1974).

Conclusions and future directions

Stuttering management therapies, including the SSMP, are based on procedures directed at desensitisation to stuttering, increasing acceptance of stuttering and motoric techniques to decrease the muscular tension associated with stuttering moments. The approaches may also include CBT. In this respect, stuttering management therapy tends to be primarily anxiolytic in emphasis (Blomgren et al., 2005).

Published treatment outcomes of the SSMP indicate that the approach does not treat stuttered speech, but rather the acceptance, avoidance, stigmatic, and anxiolytic symptoms of the stuttering disorder (Blomgren et al., 2005). Two broader conclusions from the Blomgren et al. (2005) study may be proposed. First, stuttering frequency does not appear to 'automatically' decrease in response to reductions in self-reported anxiety. In other words, decreasing anxiety alone is not sufficient to decrease stuttering frequency. However, it does appear possible to decrease anxiety related to stuttering - even in the absence of any actual decrease in stuttering frequency.

In summary, the anxiolytic aspects of stuttering do appear to be treatable, even in the absence of related decreases in stuttering frequency and severity. The positive aspects of the SSMP are in helping people who stutter manage their fears, anxieties and avoidances related to stuttering and speaking. However, it may be argued that for any stuttering treatment to be considered 'successful' the treatment should reduce stuttering frequency as well as any participation or activity restrictions (Finn et al., 2005; Yaruss, 2001; Yaruss and Quesal, 2004). Therefore, combining techniques from the SSMP with fluency shaping or speech restructuring therapies will likely result in the most extensive positive treatment outcomes.

Through research, stuttering treatment has advanced significantly over the past decade. The new standard for stuttering treatment is using combinations of treatment approaches that address overt stuttering as well as the avoidance, affective, self-perceptive and anxiolytic aspects of the disorder. However, determining the most effective combination of speech restructuring and stuttering management techniques for each stuttering speaker will likely depend on the abilities, needs and wants of the individual clients themselves. New developments in computer-aided biofeedback (Kroll and Scott-Sulsky, 2010), pharmacological treatments (Maguire et al., 2010) and self-modelling (Bray and Kehle, 1998; Prins and Ingham, 2009), combined with effective treatment maintenance strategies may also add significantly to therapy success. Identifying the essential aspects of the SSMP and perhaps combining them with other established and evidence-based treatments may lead to improved treatments all round (Blomgren, 2010).

Discussion

Joseph Attanasio

Thanks for your clear overview that provoked lots of discussion in our group. The first question I'd like to start with is why do you think this is the most common and most popular in the United States? It doesn't reduce stuttering, as you've shown. It does have obviously some impact on anxiety and some other dimensions related to anxiety, but couldn't that be achieved by other approaches such as CBT? It seems paradoxical.

Michael Blomgren

That's a very good question and of course the answer to that would just be my opinion. In the United States, not many speech pathologists use speech restructuring techniques (see Preface for a definition of this term). I would venture to say the majority of speech-language pathologists in the United States focus on stuttering management techniques. This is due to both history and the fact that the major textbooks in the United States tend to have a stuttering management emphasis to them. Also the Stuttering Foundation of America is an influential organisation that emphasises on stuttering modification.

Sheena Reilly

Your presentation prompted a lot of discussion and interest in our group as well. We were interested in what clients expect when they come to the programme.

Michael Blomgren

Generally I don't think treatment programmes advertise their intended outcomes very well. I've seen clients where I think they were expecting something quite different than what they received and that is a problem. However, I would guess that most clients come to the SSMP aware of what it's about. I would say most do their research before and know about the programme in advance. For the clients that don't know about the SSMP, it might be a bit of a rude awakening on Day 1 where they need to go out and advertise that they stutter in public. The SSMP doesn't practice systematic desensitisation; it is more like a sink or swim approach.

Joseph Attanasio

We'd like you to clarify the anxiety component here. Did you say that anxiety was reduced? Your data seemed to show that state and trait anxiety did not change.

Michael Blomgren

There wasn't a decrease with the State-Trait Anxiety Inventory but we did measure a significant post-treatment reduction for scores on the psychic anxiety and somatic anxiety subscales of the Multi-component Anxiety Inventory. We also measured a significant reduction of avoidance behaviour on the Perceptions of Stuttering Inventory. I view a reduction of avoidance behaviour to be related to anxiety.

Ann Packman

You talked about trying to identify which components of the programme might be more effective than others. Could you tell us what you think they might be? And if you were to change the design of SSMP, what changes would you make?

Michael Blomgren

The SSMP is not my programme, so any suggestions for change are purely academic. I think the dose issue is important and is currently an unknown factor. I am not sure that clients need 3 weeks to learn the SSMP techniques, so changes to the overall duration might be possible. From both a personal and a clinical perspective, I think one of the most powerful SSMP techniques is disclosure. With a little practice most clients who stutter can get into the habit of disclosing their stuttering, so I would want to emphasise that. The pseudo-stuttering technique, involving stuttering on purpose, is difficult to sell to clients. They often say, 'I came here to learn to not stutter and you're saying, "stutter more"?' So maybe the pseudo-stuttering is not as important as disclosure. The stuttering modification techniques of prolongations and pullouts can be very helpful in giving clients some skills to control the intensity of stuttering moments. My opinion is that too little time is devoted to practicing those techniques.

Sheena Reilly

We were interested in the result that there was no post-treatment move towards internal locus of control when so many of the procedures are designed to give clients control over their stuttering. Can you comment on that?

Michael Blomgren

Perhaps locus of control only changes when there is a corollary change in stuttering severity and/or perception of decreased struggle associated with stuttering. We didn't see changes in those areas in the SSMP so perhaps that is why we also didn't see post-treatment movement towards more internal locus of control. We are just completing a treatment outcome study of a comprehensive stuttering clinic that included prolonged speech techniques. We had 29 clients and we did measure a statistically significant change in locus of control (Blomgren et al., 2009). In this study, we also had a statistically significant decrease in frequency of stuttering. So perhaps decreased stuttering is necessary for a feeling of increased internal locus of control.

Joseph Attanasio

You measured changes in stuttering and recorded that stuttering frequency did not change. However, the programme helps clients modify the moment of stuttering, so what were the changes there? Were they successful in actually modifying the moment of stuttering for the better?

Michael Blomgren

That is an important question, but one for which I don't have a direct answer. We didn't specifically assess any qualitative aspects of stuttering moments, such as average duration, or amount of struggle. That is something that could certainly be done. In fact, it should be done in any future study. We have some indirect data related to your question from the scores on the SSI. The SSI provides an overall score that is based on a combination of stuttering frequency, the three longest moments of stuttering and an assessment of secondary stuttering behaviours. So, in a sense, the SSI captures some additional aspects of stuttering beyond simple frequency counts. The SSI scores did decrease significantly immediately after the treatment but the decreases were not evident 6 months later. I think a more detailed examination of how clients might be modifying moments of stuttering would be prudent.

Ann Packman

We had an interesting discussion about measuring the amount of everyday speaking. Some of your measures were to do with reading and monologues and did not tap into that. But we also discussed that, in relation to avoidance, couldn't clients reduce avoidance simply by speaking less at the end of the programme? We were interested in whether there had been any measures done on those aspects in relation to this programme?

Michael Blomgren
No.

Ann Packman
Do you think it's possible?

Michael Blomgren
Yes, it is possible, but probably somewhat difficult. One way of measuring avoidance might be to measure amount of speaking time. This could be done with a voice dosimeter. A voice dosimeter measures the speaking time per day and has been used with voice-disordered speakers. This could be an excellent real life outcome measure of stuttering treatment. I don't believe it has been used before with people who stutter.

Sheena Reilly
Our group was also interested about the satisfaction levels associated with the programme: client satisfaction of course, but also student satisfaction because it is conducted in a university clinic. How do you inform students about other treatment options for clients?

Michael Blomgren
I believe that students should receive training in a broad range of treatment options. The SSMP was offered at the University of Utah from 1998 to 2001. Our current intensive stuttering clinic is a comprehensive clinic, which replaced the SSMP in 2002. The current clinic is based on a combination of prolonged speech training and stuttering management techniques. Unfortunately, I think most university programmes in the United States teach stuttering management to the exclusion of anything else.

Sheena Reilly
That would be an innately self-reinforcing cycle favouring stuttering modification?

Michael Blomgren
Exactly.

Joseph Attanasio
You mentioned that the programme depends upon the counselling skills of the clinician. With the programme administered by students, what do they do? What does a typical day look like in terms of what students are doing with clients?

Michael Blomgren
In the SSMP, the daily routines are quite regimented. There is a 170-page manual that the clients work through. The manual has daily activities and generally the clients spend about half an hour in a group session and then meet with

their individual student clinician for about half an hour. The day progresses between group and individual sessions. Any new technique is presented in the group setting by the master clinician. The student clinicians then reinforce these techniques during individual sessions. In reality, the student clinicians are often learning the programme techniques at nearly the same time as the clients. With respect to the point about counselling, I believe many counselling issues are related to problem solving. For example, when working on disclosure a client might say, 'I'm not going to do that' or 'I can't do that'. Perhaps counselling might go along the lines of asking, 'Well, why do you think you can't do it?' or 'Exactly what would you be willing to do?' Some student clinicians get the hang of it right away and others struggle with it. As with all student supervision, it is ultimately incumbent on the clinical supervisors to help both the clients and the student clinicians acquire these skills.

Ann Packman

We wondered whether you think the programme in its current form is sustainable. The current tough economic climate[1] for people in the United States must make it difficult for clients to afford programmes like this. Considering that, and that evidence about its long-term effectiveness is limited, is SSMP viable?

Michael Blomgren

The programme has been conducted at Eastern Washington University since 1962, so history suggests it is sustainable there. On the other hand, I don't believe it is currently being offered anywhere else. The high costs associated with intensive programmes such as the SSMP do limit the amount of people that are able to attend.

Sheena Reilly

Do you have any details about clients that did better or were more satisfied with their outcomes? For example, were older clients more satisfied or clients who had, say, a speech restructuring treatment previously and then feel the need for an anxiolytic treatment?

Michael Blomgren

Participants in the SSMP have varied from young adolescents to clients in there seventies. There were clients without previous treatment history and those who had received extensive speech treatment previously. I'm not aware of any research examining these variables. Anecdotally, though, I think if a client is outgoing and willing and able to talk about their stuttering, they will likely do well in an approach such as SSMP. But I guess it's the 'avoiders' who need this type of treatment the most.

Joseph Attanasio

A statistical question for you. Your data analyses were repeated t-tests. Can we assume that these analyses contained some sort of corrections to protect against Type I errors?

---

[1]Just prior to the symposium, a global financial crisis had emanated from the United States and severely impacted the country.

Michael Blomgren

Yes, we did an adjustment procedure so the requisite significance level was small. That said, there are good arguments that it is unnecessary to make alpha adjustments in outcomes studies such as this because most measures are independent of one another. There is always a trade-off between Type I and Type II errors.

Ann Packman

We also had a discussion of what link there might be between programmes like this one, which focus on desensitisation about stuttering, and the support that people get in it by just being together, and the kind of benefits that arise from self-help groups. Could you speak a bit about what the link might be between the two?

Michael Blomgren

I think there are similarities and overlap between desensitisation programmes like the SSMP and support groups. In both cases, the process of being open to discussing stuttering and approaching speaking situations is paramount. In order for someone to even contemplate attending a self-help group, I think that there needs to be a certain level of acceptance. Acceptance of stuttering and desensitisation to stuttering are obviously linked. Indeed, clients are encouraged to join a self-help group after treatment.

References

Andrews, G., Guitar, B., & Howie, P. (1980) Meta-analysis of the effects of stuttering treatment. *Journal of Speech, and Hearing Disorders, 45*, 287–307.

Bandura, A. (1977) Self-efficacy: toward a unifying theory of behavioral change. *Psychology Review, 84*(2), 191–215.

Bandura, A. (1986) *Social Foundations of Thought and Action.* Englewood Cliffs, NJ: Prentice-Hall.

Beck, A. T., & Steer, R. D. (1993) *Beck Depression Inventory Manual.* San Antonio, TX: The Psychological Corporation.

Blomgren, M. (2010) Stuttering treatment for adults: an update on contemporary approaches. *Seminars in Speech Language, 34*(4), 272–282.

Blomgren, M., Roy, N., Callister, T., & Merrill, R. M. (2005) Intensive stuttering modification therapy: a multidimensional assessment of treatment outcomes. *Journal of Speech, Language, and Hearing Research, 48*, 509–523.

Blomgren, M., Whitchurch, M., & Metzger, E. (2009) The University of Utah Intensive Stuttering Program: Treatment Outcomes. Paper presented at the 6th World Congress on Fluency Disorders, Rio de Janeiro, Brazil.

Bloodstein, O. (1975) Stuttering as tension and fragmentation. In: J. Eisenson (Ed.), *Stuttering: A Symposium* (pp. 1–96). New York: Harper.

Bloodstein, O., & Ratner, N. B. (2008) *A Handbook on Stuttering* (6th ed.). Clifton Park, NY: Thomson/Delmar Learning.

Bothe, A. K., Davidow, J. H., Bramlett, R. E., & Ingham, R. J. (2006) Stuttering treatment research 1970–2005: I. Systematic review incorporating trial quality assessment of behavioral, cognitive, and related approaches. *American Journal of Speech-Language Pathology, 15*, 321–341.

Boudreau, L. A., & Jeffrey, C. J. (1973) Stuttering treated by desensitization. *Journal of Behavior Therapy and Experimental Psychiatry, 4*(3), 209–212.

Bray, M. A., & Kehle, T. J. (1998) Self-modeling as an intervention for stuttering. *School Psychology Review, 27*(4), 587–598.

Breitenfeld, D., & Girson, J. (1995) Efficacy of the Successful Stuttering Management Program workshops in the United States of America and South Africa. Paper presented at the First World Congress on Fluency Disorders, Nijmegen, The Netherlands.

Breitenfeldt, D. H., & Lorenz, D. R. (1999) *Successful Stuttering Management Program (SSMP): for Adolescent and Adult Stutterers* (2nd ed.). Cheney, WA: Eastern Washington University Press.

Craig, A. R., Franklin, J. A., & Andrews, G. (1984) A scale to measure locus of control of behaviour. *British Journal of Medical Psychology, 57*(2), 173–180.

Craig, A. R., & Tran, Y. (2006) Fear of speaking: Chronic anxiety and stammering. *Advances in Psychiatric Treatment, 12*, 63–68.

Crits-Cristoph, P., Baranackie, K., Kurcias, J., Beck, A., Carroll, K., Perry, K., & Zitrin, C. (1991) Meta-analysis of therapist effects in psychotherapy outcome studies. *Psychotherapy Research, 1*, 81–91.

Dalali, I. D., & Sheehan, J. G. (1974) Stuttering and assertion training. *Journal of Communication Disorders, 7*, 97–111.

De Nil, L., & Kroll, R. (1996) Therapy review: successful stuttering management program (SSMP). *Journal of Fluency Disorders, 21*, 61–64.

Dunlap, K. (1932) *Habits: Their Making and Unmaking.* New York: Liveright.

Eichstadt, A., Watt, N., & Girson, J. (1998) Evaluation of the efficacy of a stutter modification program with particular reference to two new measures of secondary behaviors and control of stuttering. *Journal of Fluency Disorders, 23*, 231–246.

Finn, P., Howard, R., & Kubala, R. (2005) Unassisted recovery from stuttering: self-perceptions of current speech behavior, attitudes, and feelings. *Journal of Fluency Disorders, 30*, 281–305.

Fishman, H. C. (1937) A study of the efficacy of negative practice as a corrective for stammering. *Journal of Speech Disorders, 2*, 67–72.

Gregory, H. (1972) An assessment of the results of stuttering therapy. *Journal of Communication Disorders, 5*, 320–334.

Ham, R. E. (1996) Therapy review: successful stuttering management program (SSMP). *Journal of Fluency Disorders, 21*, 64–67.

Howie, P. M., Tanner, S., & Andrews, G. (1981) Short- and long-term outcome in an intensive treatment program for adult stutterers. *Journal of Speech, and Hearing Disorders, 46*, 104–109.

Ingham, R. J. (1975) Operant methodology in stuttering therapy. In: J. Eisenson (Ed.), *Stuttering: A Second Symposium* (pp. 333–399). New York: Harper and Row.

Ingham, R. J. (1984) *Stuttering and Behavior Therapy: Current Status and Experimental Foundations.* San Diego, CA: College-Hill Press.

Irwin, A. (1972) The treatment and results of "easy-stammering". *British Journal of Disorders of Communication, 7*(2), 151–156.

Johnson, W. (1961) *Stuttering and What You Can Do About It.* Minneapolis, MN: University of Minnesota Press.

Johnson, W. (1967) Stuttering. In: W. J. D. Moeller (Ed.), *Speech-Handicapped School Children* (pp. 229–329). New York: Harper & Row.

Kraaimaat, F. W., Vanryckeghem, M., & Van Dam-Baggen, R. (2002) Stuttering and social anxiety. *Journal of Fluency Disorders, 27*, 319–331.

Kroll, R., & Scott-Sulsky, L. (2010) The fluency plus program: An integration of fluency shaping and cognitive restructuring procedures for adolescents and adults who stutter. In: B. Guitar & R. McCauley (Eds.), *Treatment of Stuttering: Established and Emerging Interventions* (pp. 277–311). Philadelphia: Wolters Kluwer/Lippincott Williams & Wilkins.

Kully, D., Langevin, M., & Lomheim, H. (2007) Intensive treatment of stuttering in adolescents and adults. In: E. G. Conture & R. F. Curlee (Eds.), *Stuttering and Related Disorders of Fluency* (3rd ed., pp. 213–232). New York: Thieme.

Kunz, R., & Oxman, A. (1998) The unpredictability paradox: review of empirical comparisons of randomised and non-randomised clinical trials. *British Medical Journal, 317*, 1185–1190.

Maguire, G., Franklin, D., Vatakis, N. G., Morgenshtern, E., Denko, T., Yaruss, J. S., *et al.* (2010) Exploratory randomized clinical study of pagoclone in persistent developmental stuttering: the examining pagoclone for persistent developmental stuttering study. *Journal of Clinical Psychopharmacol, 30*(1), 48–56.

Manning, W. H. (1990) Successful stuttering management program (SSMP) for adolescent and adult stutterers [Review]. *ASHA, 32*, 87–88.

Menzies, R. G., O'Brian, S., Onslow, M., Packman, A., St Clare, T., & Block, S. (2008) An experimental clinical trial of a cognitive-behavior therapy package for chronic stuttering. *Journal of Speech, Language, and Hearing Research, 51*, 1451–1464.

Menzies, R. G., Onslow, M., Packman, A., & O'Brian, S. (2009) Cognitive behavior therapy for adults who stutter: a tutorial for speech-language pathologists. *Journal of Fluency Disorders, 34*, 187–200.

Montgomery, C. S. (2006) The treatment of stuttering: from the hub to the spoke. In: N. Bernstein Ratner & J. A. Tetnowski (Eds.), *Current Issues in Stuttering Research and Practice* (pp. 159–204). Mahway, NJ: Lawrence Erlbaum.

O'Brian, S., Packman, A., & Onslow, M. (2010) The Camperdown Program. In: B. Guitar & R. McCauley (Eds.), *Treatment of Stuttering: Established and Emerging Interventions* (pp. 256–276). Philadelphia: Wolters Kluwer/Lippincott Williams & Wilkins.

Prins, D. (1970) Improvement and regression in stutterers following short-term intensive therapy. *Journal of Speech and Hearing Disorders, 35*(2), 123–135.

Prins, D., & Ingham, R. J. (2009) Evidence-based treatment and stuttering – historical perspective. *Journal of Speech, Language, and Hearing Research, 52*, 254–263.

Riley, G. (1994) *Stuttering Severity Instrument for Children and Adults.* (3rd ed.). Austin, TX: Pro-Ed.

Ryan, B. P. (1974) *Programmed Therapy for Stuttering in Children and Adults.* Springfield, IL: Thomas.

Schalling, D., Chronholm, B., Asberg, M., & Espmark, S. (1973) Ratings of psychic and somatic anxiety indicants: Interrater reliabilty and relations to personality variables. *Acta Psychiatrica Scandinavia, 49*, 353–368.

Sheehan, J. G. (1951) The modification of stuttering through non-reinforcement. *Journal of Abnormal Psychology, 46*(1), 51–63.

Sheehan, J. G. (1970) *Stuttering; Research and Therapy.* New York: Harper & Row.

Sheehan, J. (1979) Current issues on stuttering and recovery. In: H. H. Gregory (Ed.), *Controversies About Stuttering Therapy* (pp. 175–208). Baltimore, MD: University Park Press.

Spielberger, G. D., Gorusch, R. L., Lushene, R., Vagg, P., & Jacobs, G. A. (1983) *Manual for the State-Trait Anxiety Inventory (Form Y Self-Evaluation Questionnaire).* Palo Alto, CA: Consulting Psychologists Press.

Van Riper, C. (1973) *The Treatment of Stuttering.* Englewood Cliffs, NJ: Prentice-Hall.

Van Riper, C. (1986) Modification of behavior, part two. In: G. H. Shames & H. Rubin (Eds.), *Stuttering Then and Now* (pp. 367–371). Columbus, OH: Charles E Merrill Publishing Company.

Williams, D. E. (1957) A point of view about stuttering. *Journal of Speech and Hearing Disorders, 22*(3), 390–397.

Williams, D. E. (1971) Stuttering therapy for children. In: L. E. Travis (Ed.), *Handbook of Speech Pathology and Audiology* (pp. 1073–1093). Englewood Cliffs, NJ: Prentice-Hall.

Williams, D. E. (1979) A perspective on approaches to stuttering therapy. In: H. H. Gregory (Ed.), *Controversies About Stuttering Therapy.* Baltimore, MD: University Park Press.

Wolpe, J. (1958) *Psychotherapy by Reciprocal Inhibition.* Stanford, CA: Stanford University Press.

Woolf, G. (1967) The assessment of stuttering as struggle, avoidance, and expectancy. *British Journal of Disorders of Communication, 2*(2), 158–171.

Yaruss, J. S. (2001) Evaluating treatment outcomes for adults who stutter. *Journal of Communication Disorders, 34,* 163–182.

Yaruss, J. S., & Quesal, R. W. (2004) Stuttering and the international classification of functioning, disability, and health: an update. *Journal of Communicaiton Disorders, 37,* 35–52.

Zebrowski, P., & Arenas, R. M. (2011) The "Iowa Way" revisited. *Journal of Fluency Disorders, 36,* 144–157

Chapter 9

The Comprehensive Stuttering Program and Its Evidence Base

Marilyn Langevin[1] and Deborah Kully[2]

[1]University of Alberta, Montreal, AB, Canada
[2]Institute for Stuttering Treatment and Research, University of Alberta, Edmonton, AB, Canada

Overview

The Comprehensive Stuttering Program (CSP) (Boberg and Kully, 1985; Kully et al., 2007) is a treatment programme for adolescents and adults that addresses overt stuttering and the attitudinal and emotional consequences of the disorder. The CSP integrates speech restructuring (see Preface for a definition of this term) with stuttering modification to help clients reduce stuttering and manage residual stuttering. It also uses cognitive behaviour therapy methods to help clients reduce learned struggle, expectancy and avoidance behaviours and improve speech associated attitudes and confidence. Therapy is delivered in group or individual programmes at Institute for Stuttering Treatment and Research (ISTAR).

The CSP has three phases: (1) Acquisition, (2) Transfer and (3) Maintenance. The Acquisition and Transfer Phases of therapy are delivered in 3-week intensive group programmes or non-intensive individual programmes during which attendance at ISTAR is mandatory. During the Maintenance Phase of therapy clients have the option to attend group refresher programmes that are offered regularly throughout the year or they may arrange individual refresher therapy that is delivered face to face or by telehealth. Clients self-determine their needs for refresher sessions or they do so in consultation with their speech-language pathologist.

In *Acquisition*, clients learn speech restructuring, stuttering modification, cognitive behavioural techniques and self-management skills. Prolongation and other fluency-enhancing techniques, such as 'easy onsets' and 'soft contacts' are used to reduce stuttering. Prolongation rates start at approximately 40 syllables per minute (SPM) and progress to a near-normal rate of 190 ± 40

The Science and Practice of Stuttering Treatment: A Symposium, First Edition. Edited by Suzana Jelčić Jakšić and Mark Onslow.

SPM. Speech naturalness is a central focus throughout the programme. Clients receive feedback on naturalness and make their own naturalness ratings using a 10-point scale (1 = highly natural; 10 = highly unnatural). Stuttering modification skills that include cancellations, pullouts and preventative and recovery rate changes (Van Riper, 1973) are used to manage residual stuttering. In the CSP, and hereinafter in this chapter, speech restructuring and stuttering modification skills are referred to as 'fluency skills'.

Cognitive behavioural techniques include identification and re-framing of ineffective self-talk and graded exposure to feared talking situations (Webster and Poulos, 1989). During graded exposure tasks, clients systematically progress through their hierarchy of feared talking situations while using fluency skills. Cognitive-behavioural techniques are learned in large-group, small-group and individual clinician–client discussions. Discussions are supplemented by written exercises and readings that draw from *Facilitating Fluency* (Webster and Poulos, 1989). Discussion topics include managing feelings, acceptance and openness about stuttering, the use of fluency-enhancing skills, confronting avoidances, dealing with listener reactions, developing confidence, developing positive attitudes towards communication, building a supportive environment, handling regression and for adolescents, managing teasing and bullying (see Langevin et al., 2007). Regarding self-management strategies, clients learn goal setting, self-measurement, self-evaluation and problem-solving skills (Boberg and Kully, 1985; Finn, 2007; Kully et al., 2007).

During the *Transfer* Phase, clients complete standard transfer tasks, such as telephone conversations, conversations with strangers and personalised tasks, such as school, family and social talking tasks. Within each of these tasks are hierarchies of graded exposure. In this phase clients also develop self-guided speech practice plans. This prepares clients to be their own clinician during the Maintenance Phase. Preparation for development of these personalised maintenance plans begins in the Acquisition Phase but is more concentrated during the Transfer Phase.

In the *Maintenance* Phase clients carry out speech and transfer practice on their own and, as indicated previously, they access refresher therapy at the clinic when they determine that they need it. In the refresher sessions clients review the fluency skills, refine self-management skills, engage in problem solving regarding use of fluency skills and cognitive behavioural techniques and engage in transfer tasks.

Theoretical basis

As Boberg and Kully (1985) suggested, development of the CSP drew from early evidence (Adams, 1982; Boberg et al., 1983; Moore and Haynes, 1980) that stuttering results from neurophysiologically based core speech disruptions that are shaped through learning and interaction with the internal and external environment and that stuttering has psychological, emotional and behavioural sequelae. More recent brain imaging research continues to suggest a neurophysiological basis to stuttering (Brown et al., 2005; De Nil, 1999) with involvement of the basal ganglia (Alm, 2004). Thus, the CSP addresses core stuttering behaviours, feelings and thoughts associated with stuttering, and the development of positive attitudes and speech related self-confidence. As we have repeatedly stated in our earlier writings, the development of the programme drew from the work of many clinicians and researchers (e.g. see Langevin and Kully, 2003).

Demonstrated value

Since 1994, four outcome studies that obtained follow-up measures at 1-5 years post-treatment have been published. In this chapter, results of a fifth study with a new cohort provides outcomes obtained at 10 years follow-up. Prior to reviewing previously published outcomes and presenting the new 10-year follow-up results, methods that have been used in all studies will be reviewed.

Methods

In all of the studies, measures of percent syllables stuttered (%SS) and SPM were obtained from audio-recorded telephone calls that contain 2 minutes of client talk time using a button press counting and timing device. Pre-treatment and post-treatment telephone calls were made from the clinic by participants to businesses. Follow-up samples were obtained from audio-recorded surprise calls made to clients by research assistants who were not known to the clients. Clients were called at their homes or workplaces. Approximately 10 minutes of interaction time is required to obtain 2 minutes of client talk time. These methods were developed to ensure that the same amount of talk time was obtained from each participant. They were developed prior to the recommendation by Davidow et al. (2006) that speech samples should be of 3 minutes duration or contain 500 words. In Langevin et al. (2006) and Teshima et al. (2010), naturalness ratings of the follow-up speech samples were obtained using Martin et al.'s (1984) 9-point scale (1 = highly natural; 9 = highly unnatural). Fifteen-second stutter-free speech samples drawn from the follow-up speech samples were rated either by independent unsophisticated listeners (Langevin et al., 2006) or by independent sophisticated and unsophisticated listeners (Teshima et al., 2010).

In addition to analysing the follow-up speech samples to determine %SS and SPM, participants were categorised by the authors as not maintaining clinically meaningful speech gains if (1) they were not maintaining at least 50% improvement in %SS in the follow-up sample relative to their pre-treatment %SS and (2) if their follow-up measure showed regression of greater than 3 %SS relative to their immediate post-treatment %SS (see Langevin et al., 2006). Finally, self-report measures were obtained in all published studies. In Boberg and Kully (1994), the Speech Performance Questionnaire (SPQ;

adapted from Perkins, 1981) was used. The SPQ measures participants' perceptions of post-treatment speech performance. In addition to the SPQ, the remaining studies obtained self-report data using the Revised Communication Attitude Inventory (S-24; Andrews and Cutler, 1974), the Perceptions of Stuttering Inventory (PSI; Woolf, 1967) and the Self-Efficacy Scaling by Adult Stutterers (SESAS-Approach; Ornstein and Manning, 1985). The PSI measures perceptions of struggle and avoidance behaviours and expectancy to stutter. The SESAS-Approach measures confidence in approaching a variety of speaking situations.

Review of previously reported outcomes

Boberg and Kully (1994) reported on 1 and 2 years post-treatment outcomes for adults and adolescents. Langevin and Boberg (1996) reported on pre- and post-treatment outcomes for adults who had concomitant stuttering and cluttering compared to clients who had a diagnosis of stuttering only. Langevin et al. (2006) compared 1 and 2 years post-treatment outcomes for Dutch adults treated in the Netherlands with adults treated at ISTAR in Canada. More recently, Langevin et al. (2010) reported on speech and self-report outcomes and Teshima et al. (2010) reported on speech naturalness outcomes of a longitudinal study in which participants were contacted yearly for 5 years following treatment.

Regarding the 1 and 2 years outcome studies, between 71% (the Dutch group in Langevin et al., 2006) and 86% (the Canadian group in Langevin et al., 2006) of participants were categorised as maintaining clinically significant stuttering reductions. Regarding 5 year longitudinal treatment outcomes, Langevin et al. (2010) reported %SS for 1 year, 2 years, 3 years, 4 years and 5 years post-treatment. They reported that the differences between the pre-treatment and post-treatment, and the pre-treatment and 5 year post-treatment %SS measures were statistically significant and the standardised effect sizes were large. They also found that %SS measures were stable during the 5-year period. That is, no significant differences were found among the post-treatment 1–5-year measures. Eighty-three percent of the participants were categorised as maintaining clinically significant reductions in stuttering. As indicated previously, Teshima et al. (2010) reported on the naturalness ratings of the immediate post-treatment and 5-year samples. They found that the naturalness ratings improved during the post-treatment period and that the mean of the ratings for the 5-year samples was within the range of naturalness ratings given to typically fluent speakers who were age, gender and accent matched.

Langevin et al. (2010) also found statistically significant differences between the pre-treatment and 2 years post-treatment measures on the S-24, the PSI and the SESAS-Approach scale. Standardised effect sizes again were large. Because the questionnaire return rate for 3 years, 4 years and 5 years was less than 50%, data for those follow-up years were not reported. With regard to the SPQ, at 2 years post-treatment the majority of participants reported that (1) they were generally satisfied with their current speech, (2) they had the ability to use techniques to control speech most of the time or more often, (3) their confidence in their ability to speak improved and (4) they had to pay attention to speech most of the time or almost always to be fluent.

The present study: 10 years post-treatment outcomes

In this fifth study, 10-year follow-up data were obtained from 17 of 25 adults (16 men and 1 woman) who completed one of three 3-week intensive treatment programmes at ISTAR. There were no dropouts during the treatment programme. One client was excluded from the study due to concomitant mental health issues for which he was taking medication. Of the remaining seven clients for whom follow-up data could not be obtained, two were deceased and five could not be contacted due to changes in addresses and telephone numbers. Demographic data for one of the 17 participants was missing. The ages of the remaining 16 participants ranged from 18 to 54 years (mean age = 32 years). No participant reported concomitant speech, language or psychological problems. Twelve participants had received previous therapy. Ten participants had post-secondary education, five had high school education and one had completed junior high education.

Speech samples were obtained using the protocol described previously. That is, 2-minute speech samples were obtained from audio-recorded telephone calls made by participants from ISTAR to businesses at pre-treatment and post-treatment. Ten-year follow-up samples were obtained from audio-recorded surprise calls made by independent research assistants to the participants at their home or work places. The speech samples were rated by a research assistant who was independent of the study and who was trained to rate %SS and SPM using guidelines established at ISTAR for Stuttering Treatment and Research (Kully, 1986). De-identified samples from the pre-treatment, post-treatment and follow-up periods were presented in random order, thus the research assistant was blinded to the time at which the samples were collected. To determine intra-rater reliability, 10% of the data with equal representation from each measurement occasion were randomly selected to be re-rated by the research assistant. To determine inter-rater reliability, the same randomly selected samples used for determining intra-rater reliability were rated by a speech-language pathologist with expertise in stuttering who was independent of the study. Correlations for intra- and inter-rater reliabilities were 1.0 and 0.97 for %SS, respectively, and 0.95 and 0.91 for SPM, respectively. All correlations were statistically significant ($p < 0.01$).

As shown in Figure 9.1, substantial reductions in stuttering were being maintained at 10 years follow-up. A Wilcoxon signed rank test revealed a statistically significant difference between pre-treatment and 10-year measures, ($z = -3.385$; $p = 0.001$), with a large effect size ($r = 0.58$). The median %SS decreased from 8.3 %SS at pre-treatment to 1.5 %SS at 10 years follow-up. Using the procedures described previously for determining clinically meaningful reductions in stuttering, 82% of participants were categorised as maintaining

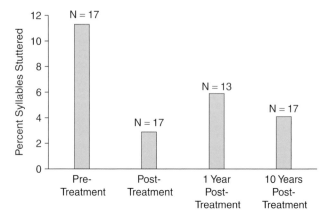

Figure 9.1 Mean percent syllables stuttered (%SS) scores for participants at pre-treatment, immediately post-treatment, 1 year post-treatment and 10 years post-treatment. Error bars are standard deviations.

clinically meaningful reductions in stuttering. The mean pre-treatment SPM was 137.3 (SD = 46.15) and the mean 10-year SPM was 152.1 (SD = 8.35). The difference between pre-treatment and 10-year SPM measures fell just short of being statistically significant (t (16) = -2.096, p = 0.052).

With regard to self-report data, S-24 pre-treatment and 10-year follow-up data were available for 10 participants and SPQ data were obtained from 12 participants at 10 years follow-up. The pre-treatment and 10-year means for the S-24 were 16.6 (SD = 5.72) and 8.5 (SD = 3.95), respectively. The difference in means was statistically significant (t (9) = 4.79) and the effect size was large (d = 1.67). With regard to the SPQ, at 10 years follow-up the majority of participants who responded reported that (1) they were generally satisfied with their current speech, (2) they had the ability to use techniques to control speech most of the time or more often, (3) their confidence in their ability to speak improved and (4) they had to pay attention to speech most of the time or almost always to be fluent.

Advantages and disadvantages

Advantages

A strength of the CSP is its integrated treatment approach in that it targets overt stuttering as well as the attitudinal and emotional consequences of the disorder. The CSP was developed to address both the overt and the psychological, attitudinal and emotional consequences of the disorder. This approach was and continues to be supported by substantial evidence of anxiety (Menzies et al., 1999) and social anxiety disorders (e.g. Menzies et al., 2008) in individuals who stutter, acknowledgement of the need to include cognitive behavioural therapy in stuttering treatment programmes (Menzies et al., 2008;

Webster and Poulos, 1989) and the need to address negative cognitions and emotions (Plexico et al., 2005).

Another strength of the CSP is its evidence base; however, there are also limitations that must be addressed in future research. Evidence of efficacy has been provided in five studies, all of which provide Phase II levels of evidence for participants in intensive treatment programmes. That is, based on Robey's (2004) five-phase model for clinical outcome research in the communication sciences, the main statistical goal of Phase II levels of evidence is to provide indications of the presence and magnitude of efficacy through point and interval estimates of effect size. The standardised effect sizes reported in the CSP studies for stuttering reductions have primarily been large, and effect sizes for improvements in perceptions of stuttering, communications attitudes and confidence have all been large.

A further strength of the CSP is the independent replication of the programme. Jehle (1995a) and colleagues delivered a German translation of the CSP to 25 clients. They reported that 71% of the 21 clients from whom measures were obtained at 8-11 weeks post-treatment were maintaining satisfactory (<3% stuttering) or marginally satisfactory (3% to <6% stuttering) outcomes. These results are comparable to 1 year outcomes reported in Boberg and Kully (1985). In contrast to Boberg and Kully (1985), Jehle (1995b) and colleagues included a refresher week and 5 refresher weekends that required attendance at the clinic. Immediately prior to the last refresher weekend 65% of the 20 clients from whom measures were obtained (Jehle, 1995a) were maintaining satisfactory or marginally satisfactory outcomes. However, as Jehle (1995a, 1995b) indicated, the group of clients treated presented with severe symptoms, with the group of clients having an average of 2.8 previous therapies and the range being 0-13 previous therapies (Jehle, 1995b).

Disadvantages

However, given the within-group effect design of these studies, the estimates of effect size are not generalisable to the population of adults who stutter who seek treatment. As well, without Phase III evidence involving a control group that receives no treatment, it is unknown whether the improvements achieved are the direct result of the CSP and what the real effect size might be in terms of an odds ratio. This limitation also applies to other speech restructuring programmes that have not yet used control group experimental designs.

A disadvantage of the CSP is that between 14% and 29% of participants across all CSP studies were categorised as not maintaining speech treatment gains. As Langevin et al. (2006, 2010) indicated, this finding is consistent with historical evidence (Craig et al., 1987; Franken et al., 1997; Howie et al., 1981) that there may be a subgroup of 20-30% of clients who are not able to maintain speech gains achieved in treatments that employ speech restructuring techniques. The reasons for these results with the CSP in particular are not yet known and warrant further investigation. It is possible that vulnerability to relapse is associated with pre-treatment stuttering severity. Pre-treatment stuttering severity measured in terms of %SS has been shown to be a weak but consistent predictor of poorer treatment outcomes (Block et al., 2006; Craig, 1998). With regard to graduates of the CSP, Huinck et al. (2006) found that participants who had more severe pre-treatment stuttering made greater gains but also suffered higher levels of relapse than those with less severe pre-treatment stuttering severity.

There is also evidence that individuals who stutter who have anxiety or other concomitant mental health disorders may be more vulnerable to relapse and may require treatment that focuses more purely on the concomitant mental health disorder (Iverach et al., 2009). Future research employing measures used by Iverach and colleagues is needed to determine the degree to which CSP clients have concomitant mental health disorders and whether or not such disorders are related to poorer CSP outcomes for individuals. If it is found that mental health disorders are predictive of poorer treatment outcomes in the CSP, then individuals who have concomitant mental health disorders may benefit from psychological treatment that is in place of or complements the cognitive-behavioural methods currently used in the programme. However, it is notable that differences between CSP participants categorised by Huinck et al. (2006) as having mild and severely negative emotional and cognitive reactions to stuttering at pre-treatment disappeared at post-treatment and at 1 and 2 years follow-up.

Other possibilities that may place individuals at risk for relapse is that the physiological basis to stuttering remains after treatment (Craig, 1998) or differences in neural plasticity exist (De Nil, 2004). It may also be that combinations of speech and attitudes (Craig, 1998; Guitar, 1976) or combinations of neuromotor, linguistic and emotional-motivational factors (McClean et al., 2004) contribute to vulnerability for relapse.

Conclusions and future directions

Across studies, including the data presented in the present report, outcomes for 135 clients treated in 3-week intensive programmes have been published. These outcomes have given Phase II levels of evidence that suggest that the CSP is efficacious in helping adolescents and adults achieve clinically meaningful and durable reductions in stuttering with speech naturalness being within normal ranges for typically fluent speakers at follow-up measures. Across five CSP studies, including the 10-year outcome data reported here, 71-86% of participants were categorised as maintaining reduced stuttering at 1, 2, 5 or 10 years post-treatment. As well, self-report data provide evidence of clinically significant improvements in communication attitudes, perceptions of stuttering and confidence in approaching speech situations.

Refinements of the CSP or development of new treatments are needed for the subgroup of clients who are not able to maintain stuttering reductions achieved in treatment with the CSP. As indicated previously, it may be that purely psychological treatments are needed in place of or in addition to the cognitive behavioural components of the CSP. Also, investigations using a comprehensive and holistic set of quantitative and qualitative measures is needed to more fully investigate the clinical significance of treatment outcomes and the process of maintenance from the perspective of clients and significant others. Finally, given the worldwide problem of limited accessibility to stuttering treatment (Carey et al., 2010; Pickering et al., 1998) there is a need to investigate the feasibility of using telehealth solely to deliver the CSP. Since 1998, ISTAR has been using telehealth to deliver refresher therapy for those adolescents and adults who complete intensive programmes and for children in non-intensive programmes (Haynes and Langevin, 2010, 2011; Kully, 2000, 2002; Loheim et al., 2011). However, given that approximately 70% of clients who come to ISTAR live outside of the two cities in which its offices are located, investigations of outcomes for treatment delivered solely through telehealth are of urgent need.

Discussion

Ann Packman

Marilyn, our group was excited by your 10 years of data and all the outcomes you measured during that period. We were interested in your definition of relapse, so could you elaborate?

Marilyn Langevin

One aspect of our determination of sustained, clinically meaningful stuttering reductions is based on percent syllables stuttered at pre-treatment relative to follow-up. In order to be considered as not being in relapse by us, that score needs to be 50% or greater. Or put another way, we consider our clients to maintain their treatment benefits if they continue have 50% stuttering improvement or more.

Ann Packman

This is not a criticism, but is that figure arbitrary?

Marilyn Langevin

It is essentially arbitrary, based to some extent on what clients tell us. If someone stutters at 60 %SS and sustains a 50 percent improvement of 30 %SS at follow-up, they will often tell us that they are doing well. Of course, this method is not perfect. For example, if someone is mild at 3 %SS pre-treatment and 2 %SS at follow-up, but has fewer of the disruptive type of stutters, then according to the criterion relapse has occurred but overall stuttering severity is less. We are trying to improve what is obviously a limited system for defining relapse. There are statistical procedures for determining clinically meaningful change that might be of value, and we are currently looking into that. One thing I didn't mention, incidentally, is that we tested for significant differences between follow-up measures 1-4 years post-treatment, to determine the stability of results, and there were no significant differences.

Joseph Attanasio

Marilyn, our group too wants to compliment you and your colleagues at ISTAR for such a commitment to evidence-based practice and the willingness of your clinicians to be part of that. One of our questions concerns the many components of the CSP. If you needed to simplify the programme, which components would you keep and which would you eliminate?

Marilyn Langevin

I would definitely keep the speech restructuring for stuttering control because obviously that's foundational. The speech pattern we use comprises 'easy breathing', 'gentle starts', 'smooth blending', which is keeping airflow moving and moving speech forward and 'light touches', which is similar to what others refer to as 'soft contacts'. If I had to trim those I think I would keep the 'smooth blending' because it incorporates breathing; you need to get air past the vocal folds in order to create sound (see Kully et al., 2007). Actually I am intrigued with the idea from Packman et al. (1994) that speech restructuring might induce acoustical changes that we have not been able to measure. I would keep the Van Riperian 'pull outs', but if I could only pick one it would be the tension reduction because although its mechanism is not clear – it might be respiratory, laryngeal, articulatory or some combination of them – it is critical for clients to reduce the tension. I think we need to retain the cognitive behavioural components, but maybe we can reduce the steps in the procedure. For those clients who are in need, I definitely would continue our referral practices to clinical psychologists who are licensed for cognitive behaviour therapy.

Sheena Reilly

Your 5–10 year outcomes look great and really promising. Can you predict the 20–30% who have poor outcomes and do you have any information about their case histories after treatment? Are they clients who have had previous treatments? Are the successful clients those who come for refresher courses?

Marilyn Langevin

The majority of adult clients who come to ISTAR have had previous treatment. We really don't know whether that helps or hinders their success in CSP. Of course, some of them have had negative treatment experiences in the past, and that certainly doesn't help. Generally with CSP the number of clients who receive refresher courses is quite small.

Sheena Reilly

Do you know how many of your participants sought other treatments during the 10-year follow-up period?

Marilyn Langevin

No, we don't unfortunately. But that of course is a well-known problem with directly determining long-term effects of speech restructuring treatments for adults. The longer the follow-up with a clinical trial, the less certain you can be that the original treatment is responsible for any observed stuttering reductions, and that is a problem that cannot really be solved with, say, a 10-year control group. The only way to really know is with an epidemiological study, and to my knowledge no such study has been published.

Ann Packman

You mentioned simplifying or shortening the cognitive behaviour therapy component. There now exists a scale that documents 66 unhelpful thoughts and beliefs about stuttering which appear to drive the social anxiety of those who stutter (Iverach et al. (2011); Clare et al. (2008)). Would that be any value for such simplification or shortening of that component?

Marilyn Langevin

I have looked at that checklist and compared it to my list of self-talk statements that have been collected over my entire career doing the cognitive behaviour therapy component of the CSP. There are few items on my list that aren't included there. I have to say I want a reduced list. So I am waiting for future simplification of that scale. Such simplification happens often during scale development. I think structural equation modelling might be a useful approach to identify factors in there, so that a 10 or 15 item scale can be developed.

Joseph Attanasio

Our group wondered how you decide who gets individual, group, intensive or non-intensive CSP treatment. Is there a screening process you use?

Marilyn Langevin

We do not have a formal screening process. We consider stuttering severity and response to clinical probes. For example, in our assessments we determine the ease with which potential clients acquire fluency skills. We also make judgments based on the type of stuttering they present with. If they are extremely tense and their breathing is severely disrupted, and if we feel that they will need all the skills we can teach, we would enrol them in the 3-week programme. On other occasions, we may wish to use an individual, non-intensive treatment programme, or even a 4-day intensive programme. We also take into account where they live. If they are living remotely, we may use the shorter intensive format then follow-up with telehealth maintenance. Telehealth technologies include interactive videoconferencing, secure web conferencing via Adobe Acrobat, Connect Pro Meeting, Skype, transmission of audio/video samples via mail or electronically and telephone calls, or a combination of these.

Sheena Reilly

We don't expect you to have an answer for this, but we think it would be a really interesting thing to reflect on. What's the way forward for conducting trials with adolescents and adults? You talked about wanting to move to a randomised controlled trial eventually. There are many independently replicated Phase I and Phase II trials of speech restructuring, and two randomised controlled trials (Carey et al., 2010; Cream et al., 2010). It seems incontrovertible that speech restructuring treatment is an efficacious method for stuttering control. So, do you think you could at present ethically conduct a trial with a no-treatment control group?

Marilyn Langevin

My view is that a randomised controlled trial could be conducted with a wait list control. We could conduct a comparison of the CSP and a modified CSP along the lines I mentioned earlier. However, I think the most pressing clinical research need for the treatment is to improve understanding of what happens in maintenance.

Sheena Reilly

Do you think no-treatment control groups are possible now? Do you think anyone would be willing to participate?

Marilyn Langevin

I think a waitlist control is feasible. But people come to ISTAR wanting treatment, so perhaps a trial with a 1-year control arm is not feasible.

Sheena Reilly

Then we get into the inadequate follow-up issue, and it becomes tricky.

Ann Packman

Marilyn, our group was interested in the ages of your clients, what is your lowest age limit and would you extend it to below that? How would you modify the CSP for young children?

Marilyn Langevin

The usual minimum age for the intensive programme is 16 years. For kids that age and 17 years it usually works for them to be with the older group of clients. With 14- and 15-year olds we will make a case-by-case decision, but we will make some modifications for their treatment, particularly with the cognitive behaviour therapy component. This involves breaking up to two groups for that treatment component during the intensive. We do treat school-age children by modifying CSP for them but retaining the essential speech restructuring components. And for that age, the cognitive behaviour therapy often needs to focus on bullying, which is of course a well-known issue for that age group.

References

Adams, M. R. (1982) Fluency, non-fluency, and stuttering in children. *Journal of Fluency Disorders, 7*, 171–185.

Alm, P. A. (2004) Stuttering and the basal ganglia circuits: a critical review of possible relations. *Journal of Communication Disorders, 37*, 325–369.

Andrews, G., & Cutler, J. (1974) Stuttering therapy: the relations between changes in symptom level and attitudes. *Journal of Speech and Hearing Disorders, 39*, 312–319.

Block, S., Onslow, M., Packman, A., & Dacakis, G. (2006) Connecting stuttering management and measurement: IV. Predictors of outcome for a behavioural treatment for stuttering. *International Journal of Language and Communication Disorders, 41,* 395–406.

Boberg, E., & Kully, D. (1985) *Comprehensive Stuttering Program.* San Diego, CA: College-Hill Press.

Boberg, E., & Kully, D. (1994) Long-term results of an intensive treatment program for adults and adolescents who stutter. *Journal of Speech and Hearing Research, 37,* 1050–1059.

Boberg, E., Yeudall, L., Schopflocher, D., & Bo-Lassen, P. (1983) The effect of an intensive behavioural program on the distribution of EEG alpha power in stutterers during the processing of verbal and visuospatial information. *Journal of Fluency Disorders, 8,* 245–263.

Brown, S., Ingham, R. J., Ingham, J. C., Laird, A. R., & Fox, P. T. (2005) Stuttered and fluent speech production: an ALE meta-analysis of functional neuroimaging studies. *Human Brain Mapping, 25,* 105–117.

Carey, B., O'Brian, S., Onslow, M., Block, S., Jones, M., & Packman, A. (2010) Randomized controlled non-inferiority trial of a telehealth treatment for chronic stuttering: the Camperdown Program. *International Journal of Language and Communication Disorders, 45,* 108–120.

Craig, A. (1998) Relapse following treatment for stuttering: a critical review and correlative data. *Journal of Fluency Disorders, 23,* 1–30.

Craig, A., Feyer, A. M., & Andrews, G. (1987) An overview of a behavioural treatment for stuttering. *Australian Psychologist, 22,* 53–62.

Cream, A., O'Brian, S., Jones, M., Block, S. Harrison, E., Lincoln, M., & Onslow, M. (2010) Randomized controlled trial of video self-modelling following speech restructuring treatment for stuttering. *Journal of Speech, Language, and Hearing Research, 53,* 887–897.

Davidow, J. H., Bothe, A. K., & Bramlett, R. E. (2006) The stuttering treatment research evaluation and assessment tool (STREAT): evaluating treatment research as part of evidence-based practice. *American Journal of Speech-Language Pathology, 15,* 126–141.

De Nil, L. (1999) Stuttering: A neurophysiological perspective. In: N. Bernstein Ratner & E. C. Healey (Eds.), *Stuttering Research and Practice: Bridging the Gap* (pp. 85–102). Mahwah, NJ: Lawrence Erlbaum Associates.

De Nil, L. (2004) Recent developments in brain imaging research in stuttering. In: B. Massen, H. F. M. Peters, R. Kent & P. H. M. M. van Lieshout (Eds.), Speech Motor Control in Normal and Disordered Speech. Proceedings of the 4th International Speech Motor Conference (pp. 150–155). Nijmegen, The Netherlands: Uitgeverij Vantilt.

Finn, P. (2007) Self-control and the management of stuttering. In: E. G. Conture & R. F. Curlee (Eds.), *Stuttering and Related Disorders of Fluency* (3rd ed., pp. 344–360). New York: Thieme.

Franken, M., Boves, L., & Peters, H. F. M. (1997) Evaluation of Dutch Precision Fluency-Shaping Program. In: E. C. Healey & H. F. M. Peters (Eds.), *International Fluency Association, 2nd World Congress on Fluency Disorders: Proceedings* (pp. 303–307). San Francisco, CA: Nijmegen University Press.

Guitar, B. (1976) Pretreatment factors associated with the outcome of stuttering therapy. *Journal of Speech and Hearing Research, 19,* 590–600.

Haynes, E., & Langevin, M. (2010) Telepractice at the Institute for Stuttering Treatment and Research (ISTAR). Paper presented at the 13th International Stuttering Awareness Day online conference for ISAD on-line forum; October. Retrieved from http://www.mnsu.edu/comdis/isad13/papers/haynes13.html

Haynes, E., & Langevin, M. (2011) Telepractice in Treating Young Children at the Institute for Stuttering Treatment and Research. Paper presented at the 9th International Stuttering Association Conference, Buenos Aires, Argentina; May.

Howie, P. M., Tanner, S., & Andrews, G. (1981) Short- and long-term outcome in an intensive treatment program for adult stutterers. *Journal of Speech and Hearing Disorders, 46*, 104-109.

Huinck, W. J., Langevin, M., Kully, D., Graamans, K., Peters, H. F., & Hulstijn, W. (2006) The relationship between the pre-treatment clinical profile and treatment outcome in an integrated stuttering program. *Journal of Fluency Disorders, 31*, 43-63.

Iverach, L., Jones, M., O'Brian, S., Block, S., Lincoln, M., Harrison, E., & Onslow, M. (2009) The relationship between mental health disorders and treatment outcomes among adults who stutter. *Journal of Fluency Disorders, 34*, 29-43.

Iverach, L., Menzies, R., Jones, M., O'Brian, S., Packman, A., & Onslow, M. (2011) Further development and validation of the unhelpful thoughts and beliefs about stuttering (UTBAS) scales: relationship to anxiety and social phobia among adults who stutter. *International Journal of Language and Communication Disorders, 46*, 286-299.

Jehle, P. (1995a) Results of the evaluation of a German version of the "Comprehensive Stuttering Program" by Boberg and Kully. In: C. W. Starkweather and H. F. M. Peters (Eds.), *Stuttering: Proceedings of the First World Congress on Fluency Disorders, Volume II* (pp. 442-444). Munich, Germany: The International Fluency Association.

Jehle, P. (1995b) Zur behandlung des stotterns mit dem therapieprogramm von Boberg und Kully - Teil 1: evaluation und kurzfristige ergebnisse. *Di Sprachheilarbeit, 40*, 385-395.

Kully, D. (1986) *Counting Guidelines.* Edmonton, Alberta: Institute for Stuttering Treatment & Research.

Kully, D. (2000) Telehealth in speech pathology: applications to the treatment of stuttering. *Journal of Telemedicine and Telecare, 6*(S2), 39-41.

Kully, D. (2002) Venturing into telehealth: Applying interactive technologies to stuttering treatment. *ASHA Leader, 7*(11). Retrieved from http://www.asha.org/Publications/leader/2002/020611/f020611_2.htm.

Kully, D., Langevin, M., & Lomheim, H. (2007) Intensive treatment of stuttering in adolescents and adults. In: E. G. Conture & R. F. Curlee (Eds.), *Stuttering and Related Disorders of Fluency* (3rd ed., pp. 213-232). New York: Thieme.

Langevin, M., & Boberg, E. (1996) Results of intensive stuttering therapy with adults who clutter and stutter. *Journal of Fluency Disorders, 21*, 315-327.

Langevin, M., & Kully, D. (2003) Evidence-based treatment of stuttering: III. Evidence-based practice in a clinical setting. *Journal of Fluency Disorders, 28*, 219-236.

Langevin, M., Huinck, W. J., Kully, D., Peters, H. F., Lomheim, H., & Tellers, M. (2006) A cross-cultural, long-term outcome evaluation of the ISTAR Comprehensive Stuttering Program across Dutch and Canadian adults who stutter. *Journal of Fluency Disorders, 31*, 229-256.

Langevin, M., Kully, D. A., & Ross-Harold, B. (2007) The Comprehensive Stuttering Program for school-age children with strategies for managing teasing and bullying. In: E. G. Conture and R. F. Curlee (Eds.), *Stuttering and Related Disorders of Fluency* (3rd ed., pp. 131-149). New York: Thieme.

Langevin, M., Kully, D., Teshima, S., Hagler, P., & Prasad, N. N. (2010) Five-year longitudinal treatment outcomes of the ISTAR Comprehensive Stuttering Program. *Journal of Fluency Disorders, 35*, 123-140.

Loheim, H., Haynes, E., & Langevin, M. (2011) Challenges and outcomes in us-ing telepractice in treating an adult from a non-western culture. Paper pre-sented at the 9th International Stuttering Association Conference, Buenos Aires, Argentina; May.

Martin, R. R., Haroldson, S. K., & Triden, K. A. (1984) Stuttering and speech natural-ness. *Journal of Speech and Hearing Disorders, 49*, 53-58.

McClean, M. D., Tasko, S. M., & Runyan, C. M. (2004) Orofacial movements associ-ated with fluent speech in persons who stutter. *Journal of Speech, Language, and Hearing Research, 47*, 294-303.

Menzies, R. G., Onslow, M., & Packman, A. (1999) Anxiety and stuttering: Exploring a complex relationship. *American Journal of Speech-Language Pathology, 8*, 3-10.

Menzies, R., O'Brian, S., Onslow, M., Packman, A., St Clare, T., & Block, S. (2008) An experimental clinical trial of a cognitive behaviour therapy package for chronic stuttering. *Journal of Speech, Language, and Hearing Research, 51*, 1451-1464.

Moore, W. H., & Haynes, W. O. (1980) Alpha hemispheric asymmetry and stuttering: some support for a segmentation dysfunction hypothesis. *Journal of Speech and Hearing Research, 23*, 229-247.

Ornstein, A., & Manning, W. (1985) Self-efficacy scaling by adult stutterers. *Journal of Communication Disorders, 18*, 313-320.

Packman, A., Onslow, M., & van Doorn, J. (1994) Prolonged speech and the modifi-cation of stuttering: perceptual, acoustic, and electroglottographic data. *Journal of Speech and Hearing Research, 37*, 724-737.

Perkins, W. H. (1981) Measurement and maintenance of fluency. In: E. Boberg (Ed.), *Maintenance of Fluency* (pp. 147-178). New York: Elsevier North Holland.

Pickering, M., McAllister, L., Hagler, P., Whitehall, T. L., Penn, C., Robertson, S. J., & McCready, V. (1998) External factors influencing the profession in six societies. *American Journal of Speech-Language Pathology, 7*, 5-17.

Plexico, L., Manning, W. H., & DiLollo, A. (2005) A phenomenological understanding of successful stuttering management. *Journal of Fluency Disorders, 30*, 1-22.

Robey, R. R. (2004) Reporting point and interval estimates of effect-size for planned contrasts: fixed within effect analyses of variance. *Journal of Fluency Disorders, 29*, 307-341.

St Clare, T., Menzies, R., Onslow, M., Packman, A., Thompson, R., & Block, S. (2008) Unhelpful thoughts and beliefs linked to social anxiety in stuttering: development of a measure. *International Journal of Language and Communication Disorders, 44*, 338-351.

Teshima, S., Langevin, M., Hagler, P., & Kully, D. (2010) Post-treatment speech naturalness of Comprehensive Stuttering Program clients and differences in ratings among listener groups. *Journal of Fluency Disorders, 35*, 44-58.

Webster, W. G., & Poulos, M. G. (1989) *Facilitating Fluency: Transfer Strategies for Adult Stuttering Treatment Programs.* Edmonton, AB: Institute for Stuttering Treatment and Research.

Woolf, G. (1967) The assessment of stuttering as struggle, avoidance and ex-pectancy. *British Journal of Disorders of Communication, 2*, 158-171.

Van Riper, C. (1973) *The Treatment of Stuttering.* Englewood cliffs, NJ: Prentice-Hall.

Chapter 10
Telehealth Treatments for Stuttering Control

Brenda Carey and Sue O'Brian
The University of Sydney, Sydney, Australia

Overview

Telehealth uses information technology and telecommunications to deliver health services to overcome treatment access barriers (Project for Rural Health Communications and Information Technology, 1996). The technologies that are used for telehealth consultations are varied, ranging from low technology options such as a standard telephone, to high technology options such as Internet teleconferencing. While it is tempting to pursue the most sophisticated technology, doing so limits accessibility. For example, virtually everyone in some societies owns a telephone and, more importantly, knows how to use it. The same is not true for Internet applications, although the number of users worldwide is increasing rapidly.

The practice of telehealth occurs in many countries, and there are several telehealth clinical trials of speech treatments for stuttering, ranging from non-randomised case studies to randomised controlled trial designs (Carey et al., 2010, in press; Harrison et al., 1999; Lewis et al., 2008; O'Brian et al., 2008; Sicotte et al., 2003; Wilson et al., 2004).

The Sicotte et al. (2003) report provided treatment with a dedicated video-conferencing suite to four children aged 3-12 years and two adolescents aged 17-19 years living remotely in Canada. However, there is no detail about which treatments were used, or whether they were used alone or combined. The authors state only that the treatments were 'currently accepted and well used procedures documented by various authors' (p. 245). They support that statement with reference to a range of classic texts by authors such as Guitar, Curlee, Van Riper and some variations of childhood treatments based on multifactorial theory (for an overview of these, see Packman and Attanasio, 2004). Additionally, the authors reported that the number of treatment hours provided to the participants was not optimal. As such, it is more

The Science and Practice of Stuttering Treatment: A Symposium, First Edition. Edited by Suzana Jelčić Jakšić and Mark Onslow.

appropriate to consider this report as an assessment of telehealth viability for child, adolescent and young adult clients, rather than a clinical trial.

There are three telehealth clinical trial reports pertaining to specific treatments: (1) the Lidcombe Program (LP; Lewis et al., 2008) and (2) the Camperdown Program (CP; Carey et al., 2010; O'Brian et al., 2008). The LP is an operant treatment designed for children younger than 6 years (Harrison and Onslow, 2010; Packman et al., 2011). The treatment guide for the LP can be downloaded from the website of the Australian Stuttering Research Centre (Packman et al., 2011). For telehealth delivery of the LP, the following adaptations were made:

(1) Treatment was by telephone.
(2) Training videotapes and written material were used.
(3) A telephone 'hotline' was made available for parents.
(4) Offline measurement of percentage stuttered syllables (%SS) and stuttering severity ratings were incorporated.
(5) Monitoring of parents doing treatment was made from audio recordings (Wilson et al., 2004).

The CP is a speech restructuring treatment designed for adults who stutter (Carey et al., 2010; O'Brian et al., 2003) that has also been adapted for use with adolescents (Carey et al., in press; Hearne et al., 2008). The generic term is 'speech restructuring' (see Preface for a definition of this term) and other common terms for treatments in this category are 'smooth speech' and 'prolonged speech'. Details of the CP are presented in Chapter 2 and the treatment manual can be downloaded from the website of the Australian Stuttering Research Centre (O'Brian et al., 2010). For telehealth delivery, the following adaptations were made:

(1) Treatment was by telephone.
(2) Client speech practice samples were forwarded to the clinician by voicemail or email.
(3) Clinician contact with clients was provided only when requested.
(4) Individual home practice replaced group practice (Carey et al., 2010; O'Brian et al., 2008).

Theoretical basis

Equity of health care is a widely accepted objective, referring to equal health care for equal need, and equal access for equal need (Turrell et al., 2006). However, in the case of people who stutter, this objective is sometimes not realised because barriers limit accessibility and availability of treatments.

In Australia, for example, people living in rural areas are disadvantaged because of clinician shortages, distance required to travel to services, unavailability of public transport and socio-economic factors (Wilson et al., 2002). People living in cities may also have difficulty accessing stuttering treatment due to long waiting lists, a shortage of clinics offering stuttering treatment programmes and, in the case of adults, practical considerations such as time away from work. For these reasons, best practice treatment cannot always be accessed.

In Australia there is a general view that the LP is best practice to treat stuttering preschool children (Harrison and Onslow, 2010). However, some service providers prohibit the provision of the weekly, hour-long treatment sessions prescribed by the programme guide (Rousseau et al., 2002). Similar difficulties are encountered in other clinical communities internationally (Pickering et al., 1998). This is concerning from the perspective of health care equity, and concerning also because the situation is likely to worsen. An aging population certainly will exacerbate future access and equity problems, as more clinicians are required to service that population.

Demonstrated value

Sicotte et al. (2003) reported client and clinician satisfaction with the telehealth treatment, but only modest %SS reductions of around 50% for the six participants, with individual results all showing clinically significant post-treatment stuttering in the range 4.0–31.5 %SS.

Lidcombe Program clinical trials

Telehealth adapted LP outcomes have been reported for three clinical trials. Harrison et al. (1999) reported that a 5-year-old boy with pre-treatment stuttering of 12–18 %SS attained the Stage 1 LP criteria after 25 telephone consultations during a 9-month period. The criteria for completing Stage 1 of the clinic LP are within-clinic %SS less than or equal to 1.0 and daily parent severity ratings of mostly 1 on a 10-point scale for 3 consecutive weeks.[1] The child in this Phase I study maintained the Stage 1 LP criteria for 23 months post-treatment. Results suggested that telehealth treatment may not have been as efficient as the in-clinic version.

Wilson et al. (2004) conducted a Phase I study with five children aged 3–5 years, again with treatment by telephone. Three pre-treatment and four post-treatment measures of %SS were collected from three 10-minute recordings at each assessment. The criteria for completion of Stage 1 were reached after 3–34 consultations. Consultations lasted between 46 and 67 minutes. Four of the five children maintained programme criteria for 12 months. Severity ratings from parents at 6 and 12 months post-treatment showed all participants were rated at severity 1–2.

Lewis et al. (2008) completed a randomised controlled trial comparing the telehealth LP with a no-treatment control arm. Twenty-two children were

---

[1]Since the conduct of the LP trials discussed here, the use of %SS during the treatment process has been deleted from the treatment manual (Packman et al., 2011). The reasons for this change are outlined by Bridgman et al. (2011).

randomised: thirteen to the control group and nine to the experimental group. All children treated with the LP achieved similar outcomes in terms of stuttering frequency to those reached in trials of the standard clinical presentation. Six of eight children in the experimental group achieved greater than 80% reduction of %SS scores, while only two of ten control children achieved similar reductions at 9 months post-randomisation.

Mean %SS scores pre-randomisation for experimental and control groups were 6.7 and 4.5, respectively. Mean %SS scores at 9 months post-randomisation for experimental and control groups were 1.1 and 1.9, respectively. Analysis of covariance adjusting for pre-randomisation severity showed a 69% stuttering decrease in the treatment group in relation to the control group. Treatment gains were maintained for up to 12 months. Parents reported high levels of satisfaction with the telehealth treatment and they confirmed that telehealth delivery did not affect rapport with the clinician. Collectively, the three studies described previously provide reasonable support for efficacy of the telehealth adapted LP.

Camperdown Program clinical trials

O'Brian et al. (2008) reported for 10 adults, aged 22–48 years, who received a telehealth adapted version of the CP by telephone. Multiple blinded outcome assessments were obtained from three 10-minute, beyond-clinic telephone conversations, one with a clinician and two from strangers. Mean pre-treatment severity was 6.9 %SS. Overall, the group achieved an 82% reduction of stuttering frequency from before treatment to immediately after treatment, and a 74% reduction of %SS from pre-treatment to 6 months post-treatment. Mean %SS post-treatment was 1.4 and at 6 months post-treatment, 1.9. Eight of the ten participants maintained their reductions up to 6 months post-treatment. Participant comments indicated that, as a group, they believed their stuttering had improved significantly and at 6 months post-treatment all still reported significant gains.

The next trial of the telehealth adapted CP was a parallel group, non-inferiority randomised controlled trial. Carey et al. (2010) compared a telephone delivered CP with the standard in-clinic version. Twenty participants were randomised to each group. As with the previous study, at no time did participants allocated to the telehealth treatment group attend the clinic. Speech outcomes involved multiple blinded assessments of %SS based on recordings of unscheduled telephone calls to participants during everyday situations. Assessments were made pre-randomisation and at 9 months post-randomisation.

The telehealth group mean %SS score pre-randomisation was 6.7 and the standard group, 5.4. At 9 months post-randomisation, the telehealth group mean %SS score was 3.0 and the standard group 2.7. The difference between the two groups was not statistically or clinically significant. Analysis of covariance adjusting for pre-randomisation severity showed that the telehealth group had 0.8 %SS lower stuttering rates at 9 months

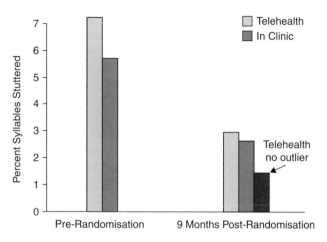

Figure 10.1 For the Carey et al. (2010) trial, mean percent syllables stuttered pre-treatment and at 9 months post-randomisation for each treatment group with, and without outlier. Used with permission from John Wiley & Sons, Ltd.

post-randomisation than the standard group (95% one-sided confidence interval 0.7% higher at most).

This effect was enhanced with the removal of data from one outlying participant, which exerted undue influence on the analyses. This participant was unique in being completely unresponsive to the treatment and retaining severe stuttering rates greater than 20.0 %SS throughout all assessments. The speech naturalness scores for both the telehealth and in-clinic groups were similar and slightly less natural than matched controls. This is a common outcome with speech restructuring treatments. Mean self-severity ratings of participants in both groups were not significantly different and confirmed the primary outcome measure. Figure 10.1 shows the mean %SS scores pre-treatment and at 9 months post-randomisation for each treatment group with and without an outlier who did not respond to treatment at all.

In terms of efficiency, the telehealth group required a mean of 10 hours 17 minutes contact time compared to the standard group mean of 12 hours 54 minutes. This difference reached statistical significance. Post-treatment questionnaires showed that while both groups expressed similar satisfaction with their treatment outcomes, the telehealth group reported the treatment by telephone was more convenient.

These two studies provide strong support for the telehealth adapted CP for three reasons: (1) both studies reported beyond-clinic, objective speech measures supported by subjective measures, (2) outcome measures were repeated and analysed independently and (3) the same procedures produced consistent outcomes.

With improvements of modern technology, the future of telehealth is likely to be Internet-based treatment, using webcam. At present we have encouraging Phase I trial results for such a version of the CP. (Carey et al., in press). Three adolescents aged 13, 14 and 15 achieved clinically significant reductions of stuttering with a mean of 11 clinician hours. The first was stuttering in beyond-clinic speaking situations pre-treatment at 16.7 %SS and at 6 months post-treatment at 1.3 %SS, but at 12 months post-treatment retained around a 50% stuttering reduction with 8.4 %SS. The other two participants fared much better. The second participant had 21.8 %SS pre-treatment, and 2.4 %SS and 2.5 %SS at 6 months and 12 months post-treatment, respectively. The third participant had 9.2 %SS pre-treatment, and 0.4 %SS and 1.6 %SS at 6 months and 12 months post-treatment, respectively.

Stand-alone Internet treatments

Perhaps the most potentially groundbreaking telehealth development is stand-alone Internet-based treatments. These treatments are completely self-directed and require no clinician input. Some progress has been made with this style of treatment with the development of a stand-alone Internet treatment and a Phase I trial of a cognitive behaviour therapy treatment for social anxiety with stuttering clients (Helgadottir et al., 2009a, 2009b). Two adult participants were no longer diagnosed with social phobia after the treatment (see Chapter 14 for details about social phobia and its treatment) and showed clinically significant improvement on a range of psychometric and quality of life measures.

There is preliminary evidence also with two participants (Erickson et al., 2012) that the CP, or some variant of it, might be viable in this format. Outcomes were measured during everyday speaking situations pre-treatment and immediately post-treatment. Participant 1 completed the programme in around 6 weeks and 26 log-ins, and Participant 2 required only 3 weeks with 35 log-ins. Participant 1 had mean pre-treatment severity of 8.7 %SS and a post-treatment mean score of 3.6 %SS. Equivalent assessments for Participant 2 were 5.6 %SS and 2.4 %SS. Both participants reported severity and situation avoidance decreased. Although these results are as yet far from compelling, and the authors reported much work to be done to refine the website, they are at least encouraging.

Advantages and disadvantages

Advantages

Telehealth stuttering treatments can contribute to equity of stuttering health care by improving access and availability of treatments. They can obviate the distance factor that prevents access by many to clinician services, and can make expert stuttering clinicians available to clients when that otherwise may not have been possible. They have the potential to provide better outcomes by means of speech restructuring techniques being learned in an everyday environment rather than a speech clinic. Although it has yet to be proven, it would not be surprising if those procedures produced more durable treatment effects because they minimise discriminated learning of stuttering control to the speech clinic and focus greater treatment responsibility on the client rather than the clinician (Stokes and Baer, 1977). A familiar treatment environment surrounded by the client's usual familial and cultural support might also be expected to promote durability of treatment effects (Bothe et al., 2006). Telehealth is far more convenient for the client, obviating the need for travel to and from the clinic during working hours and this may increase compliance and treatment continuity (Mashima et al., 2003). Finally, the overall cost of health care would be reduced by elimination of travel costs and a reduction of time away from work (Carey et al., 2010). Additionally, for clients treated with webcam Internet-based telehealth, the need for physical and personnel clinic infrastructure is obviated. And of course, if stand-alone Internet-based treatment becomes a reality, then no resources of any kind would be needed for clients to be successfully treated!

Adolescents are generally thought to be a challenging client group. There are many sources to document that they spend a great deal of time on the Internet and that it is an important focus of their social lives. Hence the advantages of Internet-based telehealth may pertain particularly to this age group. Here is what one of the adolescents said during the Carey et al. (in press) trial:[2]

> Having to do it over the Internet . . . you can choose any time in your week that you're able to do it, because if you have a set time when you have to see a person in their office . . . that can be hard on you because you have to cancel other plans for that. If you're doing it over Skype . . . it makes it very flexible so . . . you can come in contact during the week . . . I just sit in any room really but right now I'm in our TV room and just on the couch with the computer in front of me.

Disadvantages

At present a major limitation of telehealth treatment is that the evidence base is constrained by the absence of treatment trials by researchers independent of the researchers who published the original trials. Rapid development of technology with technical improvements to Internet webcams seems to be outpacing the publication of clinical trials. There are randomised controlled trials data for telehealth methods that do not involve the Internet (Carey et al., 2010; Lewis et al., 2008), but only Phase I data (Carey et al., in press) for fully Internet-based methods. It is also the case that, in contrast to standard versions of child and adult treatments, nothing is known about long-term outcomes. Although, as discussed previously, there is reason to believe that these may even be better with telehealth versions, at present it is completely an assumption that telehealth versions are even as efficacious as in-clinic versions

[2]Dr Carey showed the delegates a video interview with one of the participants in the trial, and this is a transcript of the interview.

in the long term. Finally, it is yet unknown whether the clinical community will accept and successfully implement what appears to be the inevitable tele-health method of webcam treatment. It is also quite onerous to consider the ethical aspects of telehealth stuttering treatments. The method heralds a completely new set of client confidentiality and data management issues and procedures.

Conclusions and future directions

The development of telehealth stuttering treatment is an exciting era for our profession to contemplate. Although there are no independent replications, clinical trials to date have been encouraging, and there is even a possibility of stand-alone Internet treatment being viable. If the foregoing assumptions of independent trial replications, durable long-term outcomes and clinician acceptance hold true, much about how we treat stuttering could change. The benefits of telehealth intervention are seemingly irresistible, and more so if it ever proves to be the case that stand-alone Internet treatment proves to be efficacious and viable. With evidence from the first community cohort of stuttering children ascertained prior to onset suggesting that early stuttering is far more common than previously thought (Reilly et al., 2009), telehealth intervention may be particularly important to handle the health care problems it poses. With the rapid advances of Internet technology, it may even be worth contemplating an era when professional preparation methods, and standard intervention methods for children and adults, are Internet based, and in-clinic treatment becomes an unusual service delivery model.

Discussion

Ann Packman
Our group was interested in variation of responsiveness to telehealth presen-tation of the CP for adults. Do you have any idea about what might predict how well people respond to it compared to standard treatment?

Brenda Carey
During the randomised control trial (Carey et al., 2010), the only predictor of post-treatment stuttering severity was pre-treatment stuttering severity. Previous treatment appeared to have no influence, nor did gender or family history. The trial was randomised, so we thought that participants who did not want the telehealth treatment and preferred the clinic version, but were randomised to telehealth, would not do as well, perhaps because they were technology shy. But results showed that not to be the case. The telehealth group did just as well, in fact better with the outlying participant removed, and they evaluated the treatment a little more positively, particularly in terms of convenience.

Ann Packman

Tell us about that outlying participant.

Brenda Carey

His stuttering was extremely severe, and although he had previously participated in three intensive speech programmes, he had not responded well to those. He was compliant but speech restructuring treatment just wasn't helpful for him.

Joseph Attanasio

Brenda could you tell us why you think that clinician-free treatment is an aspiration? And what might the risks be?

Brenda Carey

Yes, I didn't think that would be a popular thing to say to a group of clinicians when it conceivably foreshadows being out of a job. I think if you put it in the context of stepped care it is not such an onerous prospect.[3] If the simplest intervention is stand-alone Internet treatment, and it mops up the health care needs of even a few of our clients, that would be a wonderful thing. Who knows, such a treatment mode may be way more successful than that.

Sheena Reilly

Brenda, someone in our group shared with us an experience working with some adolescents who felt that using webcam actually made them much more fluent. It was a medium that they often chose, for example, if talking to a girlfriend. So our question is could webcam itself act as a discriminative stimulus for stutter-free speech, considering what you talked to us about today?

Brenda Carey

I have thought about that. Participants, particularly adolescents, are at their computers often and they do a lot of talking, socialising, even shopping around their computers. So I would not be surprised if you are correct. So, if discriminated learning of stuttering control does occur with the Internet, then that would be far less of an evil than discriminated learning occurring within a clinic. The critical point here in what you say underscores the importance of having outcome measures for Internet telehealth trials independent of the Internet.

Ann Packman

Our group was interested in the interaction that occurs during the LP when you do it with webcam. How does the child really like seeing you on webcam? Do children feel that someone is actually talking to them? How do you interact with the parent? Is it like a standard session in the clinic?

Brenda Carey

So far the trials that have been done have been on LP, delivered over the phone only, but it is true that a randomised controlled trial is underway with

---

[3]The stepped care model of health care is overviewed in Chapter 4, p. 49.

a collaboration between the Australian Stuttering Research Centre in Sydney and La Trobe University in Melbourne. That trial compares webcam LP with the standard, in-clinic version. The children are face to face with the clinician for at least part of the session and will look very much like a child appears during a clinic session. I have had experience with webcam treatment and I find that there is little problem with establishing the usual clinical rapport with child or parent over the Internet, particularly with image and audio quality improving with technology every year.

Joseph Attanasio

Brenda, does Speech Pathology Australia have ethical guidelines for telehealth treatment, or are there moves towards developing them? In the United States, the American Speech-Hearing Association has developed some pretty strict guidelines for telehealth.

Brenda Carey

Not yet, it is early days in Australia in terms of issues such as ethics and health fund rebates and incorporation of telehealth into public health services for stuttering.

Sheena Reilly

Just a comment before a question. In our group we had the same discussion about regulation and Marilyn Langevin tells us that one province in Canada has refused permission for telehealth to occur across provinces. Now to our question. You said with reference to stepped care that telehealth may not be for all clients who stutter. Who do you think it is not for? We had a discussion about which parents and which children this might not suit, so could you address that with particular reference to age groups.

Brenda Carey

For treating children with the LP, telehealth would not be recommended as a first treatment of choice because it does take longer in the low-tech version so far tested. Webcam trials may reveal different findings, but for now we just do not know. For now if it is easy enough for a parent to get to a clinic, then for the preschool-age group I would suggest clinic-based treatment. For adolescents and adults, the existing evidence gives a different picture. For them, telehealth treatment is looking more efficient than in-clinic treatment, so if it is cheaper and easier and takes fewer hours, why would we not recommend it for any or adolescent or adult? So I am pretty open to using it for any adolescent or adult who would prefer it. There are adults who are able to continue their normal workday by fitting in their speech therapy over lunch or at a 7.30 am appointment, or who travel to different countries and can have their sessions from there. Such treatment continuity that is possible with telehealth is a big plus.

Ann Packman

Brenda this is just a request for clarification about the different models of the telehealth delivery method: the teleconferencing suite, the telephone and webcam.

Brenda Carey

We just use a normal telephone. A mobile phone can be used, but of course it is more expensive for conducting a clinical trial. For the webcam trials I just mentioned, they are using a programme which is free and can be downloaded by anyone anywhere in the world and that requires client and clinician to have a webcam and a microphone. Conveniently, most laptops these days have both. Regarding videoconferencing, a remotely located suite was used with the Sicotte et al. (2003) trial, but with the rapid proliferation of webcam, at least for stuttering treatment, it generally seems a redundant technology. Unless, of course, there are places in the world where Internet access for various reasons is not available and a videoconferencing suite is.

Ann Packman

I think maybe in Canada, where the Sicotte et al. (2003) trial was conducted, teleconferencing suites are used.

Marilyn Langevin [From the floor]

That is true. At least in Alberta such suites exist at public health centres. But in a sense they counteract the access advantages of telehealth, because clients and their parents need to go to those suites.

Joseph Attanasio

Brenda, on the issue of efficiency, could you comment about the difference between convenience and efficiency. Do you agree that we need to be aware of the distinction when reporting treatment efficiency data?

Brenda Carey

Absolutely. In all of the studies I discussed today, with the exception of the Sicotte et al. (2003) study, there are reports of clinician contact time, which is efficiency, while other data from post-treatment questionnaires pertain to convenience, or client satisfaction. Such questionnaires typically use scales to elicit from clients information related to satisfaction: how convenient they found the treatment, how easy it was to fit into their lives, how easy was it to get to know the clinician, and so on.

Sheena Reilly

Brenda, in your experience so far, do you think parents of stuttering children behave as naturally when they are involved in a webcam treatment as they do in a clinic?

Brenda Carey

Again, since there's no data about this, I can just give my impression from my current clinical work. Definitely, I think parents feel more relaxed with webcam, as do adults and adolescents. My feeling is that people attending a clinic, whether it is a medical centre or a dental surgery or a physiotherapy clinic, experience some disempowerment in those environments. At home they are more relaxed and I think that possibly aids what they need to learn, whether it be as parents of stuttering children or clients themselves.

Ann Packman

We had some discussion about determining the appointments, if you like to call them that. When you are doing LP or CP with webcam, did you do it on a weekly basis, as occurs with the in-clinic versions?

Brenda Carey

They were both exactly as would have occurred with in-clinic treatments. People missed appointments sometimes due to being sick or on holidays or whatever. Overall, the intention has been to follow the treatment manuals as closely as possible. In fact, in some respects it was easier to maintain treatment continuity with webcam, as I said before. Minor illness or travel that would prevent in-clinic treatment sessions would not necessarily have the same effect on webcam sessions.

Joseph Attanasio

Brenda, have you found any webcam differences with how you administer treatment between LP and CP? We were wondering because the clinician has a completely different role with the two treatments; with the former the clinician teaches the parent how to do the treatment with the child but with the latter shows the adult directly what to do.

Brenda Carey

There are differences of course. With webcam you need to work differently when you are looking at a scene of a parent and child at home and you have to model how to do the treatment and look at the parent doing it over webcam. The procedure is different to in-clinic LP. But with the CP I see no difference at all with how the treatment is presented.

Sheena Reilly

I just want to come back to Joseph's earlier point about cautions with a possible transition to Internet-based, clinician-free treatments. Our group wanted to know whether the treatments will be just reading material, and that after reading it parents and clients simply apply the recommendations to themselves as they see fit?

Brenda Carey

Definitely not. The promise of the stand-alone Internet treatments for cognitive behaviour therapy I mentioned (Helgadottir et al., 2009a, 2009b) seems to be related to a number of important factors. One is individualisation of the treatment to the specific needs of the client based on online assessment, and the capacity of the programme to generate large numbers of treatment activities based on that assessment. 'One size fits all' clearly cannot happen with any kind of stuttering treatment, either Internet driven or otherwise.[4]

---

[4]The Internet program in question (CBTPsych.com) also attempts to create the feel of a 'real' therapist with recordings and images of real clinicians who explain the treatment and guide clients through it. Although those who attempt to use speech restructuring treatments to control stuttering encounter a great many problems to solve, they are nonetheless finite in number and can be taken account of with stand-alone Internet treatment development.

Ann Packman

Can you give us any more details about the clinical trial under way of in-clinic LP compared with webcam LP?

Brenda Carey

It is for children younger than 6 years and it is a randomised controlled non-inferiority trial.

Joseph Attanasio

Brenda you alluded to this before, but I would like a direct assessment if you could about how the webcam telehealth mode affects developing a clinician/client relationship. Is there a difference? Does it take longer?

Brenda Carey

I think as clinicians we are all anxious about this aspect of the treatment development. But I have found very little difference at all: not with parents and not with adolescent clients. I think that many clients will demand telehealth treatment in the future, and I know that many are already demanding it. I think that we need to get past an assumption that in-clinic face-to-face contact is superior to webcam face-to-face contact in terms of rapport. Let's not forget that both modes are face-to-face. I am not sure whether that is an empirical question or whether it is self-evident. It certainly is self-evident to me based on my experience, but of course, during clinical trials, secondary outcome variables about this dimension of the treatment would probably be a good idea.

References

Bothe, A. K., Davidow, J. H., Bramlett, R. E., & Ingham, R. J. (2006) Stuttering treatment research 1970–2005: I. Systematic review incorporating trial quality assessment of behavioral, cognitive, and related approaches. *American Journal of Speech-Language Pathology, 15*, 321–341.

Bridgman, K., Onslow, M., O'Brian, S., Block, S., & Jones, M. (2011) Changes to stuttering measurement during the Lidcombe Program treatment process. *Asia Pacific Journal of Speech, Language, and Hearing, 14*, 147–152.

Carey, B., O'Brian S., Onslow, M., Block, S., Jones, M., & Packman, A. (2010) Randomised controlled non-inferiority trial of a telehealth treatment for chronic stuttering: the Camperdown Program. *International Journal of Language and Communication Disorders, 45*, 108–120.

Carey, B., O'Brian, S., Onslow, M., Packman, A., & Menzies, R. (in press) Webcam delivery of the Camperdown Program for adolescents who stutter: a Phase I trial. Language, Speech, and Hearing Services in Schools.

Erickson, S., Block, S., Menzies, R., Onslow, M., O'Brian, S., & Packman, A. (2012) Standalone Internet speech restructuring treatment for adults who stutter: a Phase I trial. Manuscript in preparation.

Harrison, L., & Onslow, M. (2010) The Lidcombe Program for preschool children who stutter. In: B. Guitar & R. McCauley (Eds.), *Stuttering Treatment: Established and Emerging Approaches.* Baltimore, MD: Lippincott Williams and Wilkins.

Harrison, E., Wilson, L., & Onslow, M. (1999) Distance intervention for early stuttering with the Lidcombe Programme. *Advances in Speech Language Pathology, 1*, 31–36.

Hearne, A., Packman, A., Onslow, M., & O'Brian, S. (2008) Developing treatments for adolescents who stutter: a Phase I trial of the Camperdown Program. *Language, Speech, and Hearing Services in Schools, 39,* 487–497.

Helgadottir, F. D., Menzies, R. G., Onslow, M., Packman, A., & O'Brian, S. (2009a) Online CBT II: a Phase I trial of a standalone, online CBT treatment program for social anxiety in stuttering. *Behaviour Change, 26,* 254–270.

Helgadottir, F. D., Menzies, R. G., Onslow, M., Packman, A., & O'Brian, S. (2009b) Online CBT I: bridging the gap between Eliza and modern online CBT treatment packages. *Behaviour Change, 26,* 245–253.

Lewis, C., Onslow, M., Packman, A., Jones, M., & Simpson, J. A. (2008) Phase II trial of telehealth delivery of the Lidcombe Program of Early Stuttering Intervention. *American Journal of Speech-Language Pathology, 17,* 139–149.

Mashima, P. A., Birkmire-Peters, D. P., Syms, M. J., Holtel, M. R., Lawrence, P. A., Burgess, L. P. A., Peters, L. J. (2003) Telehealth: voice therapy using telecommunications technology. *American Journal of Speech-Language Pathology, 12,* 432–439.

O'Brian, S., Carey, B., Onslow, M., Packman, A., & Cream, A. (2010) The Camperdown Program for stuttering: treatment manual. Retrieved from http://sydney.edu.au/health_sciences/asrc/docs/camperdown_manual.pdf

O'Brian, S., Onslow, M., Cream, A., & Packman, A. (2003) The Camperdown Program: Outcomes of a new prolonged-speech treatment model. *Journal of Speech, Language, and Hearing Research, 46,* 933–946.

O'Brian, S., Packman, A., & Onslow, M. (2008) Telehealth delivery of the Camperdown Program for adults who stutter. *Journal of Speech, Language, and Hearing Research, 51,* 184–195.

Packman, A., & Attanasio, J. S. (2004) *Theoretical Issues in Stuttering* (1st ed.). New York: Taylor & Francis.

Packman, A., Onslow, M., Webber, M., Harrison, E., Lees, S., Bridgeman, K., & Carey, B. (2011) The Lidcombe Program of early stuttering intervention treatment guide. Retrieved from http://sydney.edu.au/health_sciences/asrc/docs/lp_manual_2011.pdf

Pickering, M., McAllister, L., Hagler, P., Whitehill, T. L., Penn, C., Robertson, S. J., & McCready, V. (1998) External factors influencing the profession in six societies. *American Journal of Speech-Language Pathology, 7,* 5–17.

Project for Rural Health Communications and Information Technology. (1996) *Telehealth in Rural and Remote Australia.* Moe, Victoria, Australia: Australian Rural Health Research Institute, Monash University.

Reilly, S., Onslow, M., Packman, A., Wake, M., Bavin, E. L., Prior, M., Eadie, P., Cini, C., Bolzonello, C., & Ukoumunne, O. C. (2009) Predicting stuttering onset by the age of 3 years: a prospective, community cohort study. *Pediatrics, 123,* 270–277.

Rousseau, I., Packman, A., Onslow, M., Dredge, R., & Harrison, E. (2002) Australian speech pathologists' use of the Lidcombe Program of early stuttering intervention. *Acquiring Knowledge in Speech, Language and Hearing, 4,* 67–71.

Sicotte, C., Lehoux, P., Fortier-Blanc, J., & Leblanc, Y. (2003) Feasibility and outcome evaluation of a telemedicine application in speech-language pathology. *Journal of Telemedicine and Telecare, 9,* 253–258.

Stokes, T., & Baer, D. (1977) An implicit technology of generalization. *Journal of Applied Behavior Analysis, 10,* 349–367.

Turrell, G., Stanley, L., deLooper, M., & Oldenburg, B. (2006) Health inequalities in Australia: morbidity, health behaviours, risk factors and health service use [Electronic Version]. Retrieved from http://www.aihw.gov.au/publications/index.cfm/title/10272.

Wilson, L., Lincoln, M., & Onslow, M. (2002) Availability, access, and quality of care: inequities in rural speech pathology services and a model for redress. *Advances in Speech-Language Pathology, 4*, 9-22.

Wilson, L., Onslow, M., & Lincoln, M. (2004) Telehealth adaptation of the Lidcombe Program of Early Stuttering Intervention: five case studies. *American Journal of Speech-Language Pathology, 13*, 81-93.

Chapter 11

A Multidimensional, Integrated, Differentiated, Art-Mediated Stuttering Programme

D. Tomaiuoli[1], F. Del Gado[2], E. Lucchini[1] and M. G. Spinetti[2]

[1]University of Rome, La Sapienza, Rome, Italy
[2]CRC Balbuzie, Rome, Italy

Overview

Our Multidimensional, Integrated, Differentiated, Art-Mediated Stuttering Programme (the MIDA-SP) is tailored to the specific needs of clients. The basic elements of each treatment are duration, intensity and structure. These elements are determined for each client by three factors. The first is the stuttering characteristics determined from the client assessment. This is the main determinant of the type of treatment presented. The second factor is the client's age, which determines the type of therapy activities chosen for them. Children and adolescents will have an intervention that also includes their parents and teachers through counselling. The third factor that determines the duration, intensity and structure of treatment is the client's expectation.

The assessment takes account of both the covert and overt aspects of the disorder and involves the following components: (1) fluency assessment, (2) assessment of the communicative behaviour and of the attitude towards stuttering, (3) linguistic assessment, (4) cognitive assessment, (5) personality assessment, (6) for children and adolescents, information about environmental factors obtained by interviews with parents and teachers and (7) general motivation for treatment displayed by the client.

The Science and Practice of Stuttering Treatment: A Symposium, First Edition. Edited by Suzana Jelčić Jakšić and Mark Onslow.
© 2012 John Wiley & Sons, Ltd. Published 2012 by John Wiley & Sons, Ltd.

The assessment tools are Systematic Disfluency Analysis (Campbell and Hill, 1999)[1] to evaluate fluency, and the following test battery: (1) Overall Assessment of the Speaker's Experience of Stuttering (OASES; Yaruss and Quesal, 2006) or the version for children Assessment of the Child's Experience of Stuttering (ACES; Yaruss et al., 2006),[2] (2) the Perceptions of Stuttering Inventory (PSI; Woolf, 1967), (3) a scale to measure Locus of Control of Behaviour (Craig et al., 1984) and (4) the modified Erickson Scale of Communication Attitudes (S-24; Andrews and Cutler, 1974).

The MIDA-SP approach provides clients with different activities, designed to work on both the overt and covert aspects of their stuttering. The goal of our therapy is to reduce the levels of both. The programme is a combination of modules offering different activities – speech therapy, transfer activities and art-mediated training – as discussed in the following text. Some activities occur in individual sessions, others in group ones.

Speech therapy

This comprises exercises to: (1) train the client to relieve muscle tension and attain correct coordination of breathing, phonation and articulation, (2) teach the client fluency-enhancing techniques and (3) teach the client fluency shaping techniques.

Transfer activities

These are designed to desensitise clients to difficult speech situations feared and avoided by clients. Therapy activities are: (1) use of the telephone, (2) conversation, (3) public speaking, (4) simulations of daily living, (5) role playing of situations and (6) participating in activities beyond the clinic. These activities allow clients to use fluency-enhancing techniques learned during therapy sessions and train them to manage different situations, reducing tension and reactions of avoidance of them.

Art-mediated training

The MIDA-SP is a combination of live theatre performance by clients (Tomaiuoli, 2005), the dubbing of client voices into movies (Tomaiuoli et al., 2006) and performed reading of tales (Tomaiuoli et al., 2009).[3] The uniqueness of art-mediated training is in giving clients activities that are far from

---

[1]This report is not published but is available to readers on request from the first author of this chapter at crc.balbuzie@tiscali.it.
[2]The OASES is now published by Pearson Assessments as three separate versions for children, adolescents and adults.
[3]This report is not published but is available to readers on request from the first author of this chapter at crc.balbuzie@tiscali.it.

their usual experiences and hence, are challenging for them. The use of the arts is intended to make the treatment more motivating and stimulating. The activities are introduced gradually, through increasing levels of difficulty, in order to encourage the use and the generalisation of both fluency-enhancing and breathing techniques. There are three stages of art-mediated training: (1) the client experiences them within a group of peers (2) the client is supported and guided, being able to restate thoughts and sensations during individual speech therapy sessions and (3) the therapist receives feedback from an art-mediated theatre trainer regarding the client responses.

These activities are designed to create positive experiences, which can eliminate the client's cognitive distortions, increase their exposure to feared situations and train clients to better manage them. A certain type of art-mediated training can be more effective in the treatment of some aspects of stuttering. In our experience, theatre is the best-suited activity for clients who display moderate to severe covert stuttering features. For adolescents and adults, dubbing of their voices into movies is best, and for children performed reading is best. Each client performs an activity with personalised goals, based on their profile, age and needs. The therapeutic goals are defined and re-elaborated by the client together with the therapist during individual therapy sessions. In those individual sessions clients report their feedback and are monitored by therapists.

Theoretical basis

MIDA-SP relies upon two conceptual premises. The first is that stuttering is viewed as a multifactorial disorder (Cook and Rustin, 1997; Gregory, 2003; Smith and Kelly, 1997; Van Riper, 1982; Yairi, 2007). As Smith and Kelly (1997) write, 'stuttering emerges from the complex, non-linear interaction of many factors' (p.209). This produces 'a multifactorial framework incorporating physiological, linguistic, environmental and psychological components' (Cook and Rustin, 1997, p.251).

The second conceptual premise is that the complex interaction among different factors at the basis of stuttering can be different from person to person. As Yairi (2007) states: 'the disorder's vast richness of overt and covert characteristics and their very diverse presence in individual stuttering patterns have been recognised for many years' (p. 168). This implies that stuttering can assume different forms in different persons affected by it.

From these premises, we can say that just as stuttering assessment has to be comprehensive and multidimensional, the same applies to the treatment, which has to be multidimensional, integrated (Starkweather and Givens-Ackerman, 1997) and differentiated for each person who stutters. From our assessment of overt and covert stuttering features, each client can be categorised (see Hicks, 2005) to establish a profile for each client. We identify four different profiles, as presented in Table 11.1.

Table 11.1 Four client profiles based on categorisation of their overt and covert stuttering features as mild or moderate to severe.

		Covert features	
		Mild	Moderate to severe
Overt features	Mild	Profile A	Profile B
	Moderate to severe	Profile C	Profile D

Profile A: Mild overt and mild covert features

The duration of treatment for clients with Profile A is $5\frac{1}{2}$ months and requires 44 hours of treatment. Clients of this type are often children and adolescents brought to therapy by anxious parents. The goals for this kind of client are to reduce overt aspects of stuttering and, at the same time, in the case of children, to let their parents learn about and understand the disorder. This can help them develop a holistic understanding of their children, beyond their stuttering. Clients first undergo a 2-month period of individual speech therapy sessions. After that, they undergo a second period of therapy that lasts $3\frac{1}{2}$ months, which is accompanied by transfer activities. They do not undertake any art-mediated training.

Profile B: Mild overt and moderate to severe covert features

The duration of treatment for clients with Profile B is 12 months and requires 102 hours of treatment. This type of client is extremely anxious about their social presentation and possible negative consequences of their stuttering. Therefore, the treatment has several goals: (1) to increase knowledge and awareness of the disorder, (2) to increase the number and type of speaking situations into which they enter and (3) to modify avoidance behaviours and improve both assertiveness and self-esteem. Group activities are particularly important for clients with this profile. During the first 2 months of treatment clients undergo an intensive series of individual therapy sessions. Subsequently, individual weekly therapy occurs for $6\frac{1}{2}$ months. Transfer activities occur starting from the third month until the end of the programme. Art-mediated training occurs from $5\frac{1}{2}$ months onwards and lasts 5 months. Clients undergo an art-mediated training specifically for their profile.

Profile C: Moderate to severe overt and mild covert features

The duration of treatment for clients with Profile C is 12 months and requires 110 hours of treatment. This type of client does not display any particular problems dealing with stuttering, even though the overt aspects of their stuttering are not mild. For this reason, the goals for their treatment focus on overt aspects of stuttering and providing them with effective behavioural tools that enable them to best manage their speech. Clients first undergo 4 months of individual treatment, focused on speech control. From this point onwards, individual sessions will support the programme once a week for $6\frac{1}{2}$ months. Clients undergo transfer activities after the first 4 months until the end of the programme. Art-mediated training is scheduled from $5\frac{1}{2}$ months and for 5 months subsequently. The art-mediated training for this type of client is movie dubbing for adults and adolescents and performed reading for pre-adolescents and children.

Profile D: Moderate to severe overt and covert aspects

The duration of treatment for clients with Profile D is 12 months and requires 124 hours of treatment. This type of client displays high levels of both dimensions of stuttering. For this reason, the goals of the therapeutic intervention are: (1) reduction of overt aspects, (2) transfer of fluency-enhancing techniques, (3) facilitating natural generalisation of these techniques and (4) reduction of avoidance reactions. Clients first undergo 2 months individual therapy, focused on speech control. From this point onwards, individual weekly sessions occur. From the third month until the end of the programme the clients undergo transfer activities. After $5\frac{1}{2}$ months from the start of their treatment, for 5 months they attend art-mediated training.

After clients complete their treatment, they are monitored during a follow-up period every 6 months for 2 years. This follow-up monitors both overt and covert stuttering features.

Demonstrated value

Tomaiuoli et al. (2006) published a file audit report of the outcomes of 'a 12 months rehabilitation programme for disfluency integrating logopedic therapy and art therapy' (p. 460) specifically consisting of movie-dubbing with 10 adults. Participants were tested just before the start of the treatment, 12 months later (when they had completed the 'logopedic therapy and art therapy') and 5 months later (when they had completed the dubbing component). Using the method of Campbell and Hill (1999), there was a reduction of 68% in the number of stuttered words from the first assessment to the final assessment around 18 months later. The participants were tested also with an adaptation of Schindler's (1980) self-evaluation of verbal conditions. Mean scores on the Avoidance component of Schindler's self-evaluation and on the Emotional Reactions component from the first to the last assessment showed a reduction of about 45%. Participants also were tested with Spielberger's (1983) State-Trait Anxiety Inventory, just before the dubbing component began and

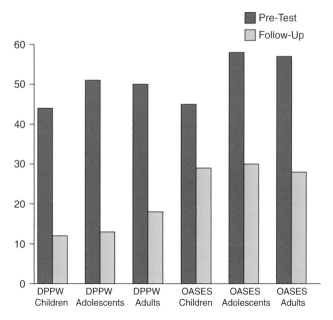

Figure 11.1 Mean pre-treatment and follow-up file audit data. DPPW, disfluencies per pronounced words; ACES, Assessment of the Child's Experience of Stuttering; OASES, Overall Assessment of the Speaker's Experience of Stuttering.

just before competing the last of the dubbing sessions. Results showed a 31% reduction.

In the following text, we present data from a file audit of 153 of our clients. Figure 11.1 presents data from our standard clinical assessments (see Overview) using the Systematic Disfluency Analysis (Campbell and Hill, 1999)[4] of within-clinic speech. Clients were treated for 12 months, and then follow-up assessment took place about 6 months later. The data presented in Figure 11.1 are pre-treatment and follow-up means of the reading, monologue and conversation tasks for number of stuttered words from a 200-word sample. Figure 11.1 shows a 70% improvement of overt stuttering features. Results for children and adolescents were similar at 73% and 75% improvement, respectively, while reported a 64% improvement for adults in the sample.

Figure 11.1 also presents covert stuttering features pre-treatment and follow-up measured with the standard OASES (Yaruss and Quesal, 2006) or the version for children ACES (Yaruss et al., 2006). Figure 11.1 shows a 46% improvement of covert stuttering features. It is not shown in the graph, but improvement scores for children, adolescents and adults were, respectively, 35%, 49% and 51%.

---

[4]This report is not published but is available to readers on request from the first author of this chapter at crc.balbuzie@tiscali.it.

Advantages and disadvantages

Advantages

The primary advantage of the MIDA-SP approach is that it provides an integrated and parallel approach to the overt and covert features of stuttering. It exposes clients to novel experiences, offering a stimulating and motivating approach to therapy. We believe that such a multidimensional approach favours the generalisation of acquired skills into everyday life. The treatment combines standard methods and methods personalised for individual clients.

Disadvantages

The disadvantages of the MIDA-SP programme are: (1) the long time it involves and (2) the related costs. In the case of children and adolescents who stutter, these costs are added to by clinician efforts to engage their parents.

Conclusions and future directions

During many years of administration and file audit testing, the MIDA-SP programme has appeared to be effective in consistently reducing both overt and covert aspects of stuttering. The treatment has been shown to favour the personal growth of the person who stutters using a holistic perspective. The programme format presented here is the result of many years spent working on its design, testing and refinement.

The next step will be its further refinement and evidence-based assessment. We plan that future research will reduce the duration and the cost of the programme but at the same time will preserve its effectiveness. We are studying two possible future treatment formats: a single period of therapy, shorter than the present, or a sequence of several shortened therapy periods.

Discussion

Mark Onslow
While the discussion groups were convening, the observers (see Preface for an explanation of who the observers were) watched some videos that we would like to play for the entire group. Francesca, could you explain the content of these videos briefly before showing them?

Francesca Del Gado
This is a short video about dubbing, which is an art-mediated training part of our programme, as we said. It allows us to expose clients to a favourite situation, but under time pressure. In fact, dubbing requires them to say specific words at a specific time during the movie track. In this way, clients can

practice the use of breathing techniques, as well as fluency-enhancing and shaping techniques. Clients learn to express emotions through their voices and learn to modulate their voices in different ways. After that, they can say, 'Well, I gave my voice to Robert De Niro!'

Now you will see one client who is trying to synchronise his speech with what Robert De Niro is saying in 'The Godfather'. And here is a segment of that movie dubbed by a client.

Joseph Attanasio

Could you explain how you came upon the idea to use dubbing in your programme?

Francesca Del Gado

The ideas I am honoured to describe are Donatella Tomaiuoli's ideas.

Joseph Attanasio

Could you also explain a bit more about what is involved in theatre?

Francesca Del Gado

We believe in the need to work on both overt and covert features of stuttering. Art-mediated training such as dubbing or theatre, or performed reading of tales, is useful to work effectively on both aspects of stuttering. This kind of approach is extremely versatile and gives the clinician a chance to personalise goals for each client's needs. For example, if I know that the client has a particular difficulty with starting the first syllable of the first word, I can ask that client to dub a part of a movie that has a great deal of dialogue (and so many starts) to help overcome that problem. An important difference between using dubbing and theatre performance is that the latter enables clients to use their bodies as a nonverbal communication tool.

Joseph Attanasio

And for how long have you been doing this?

Francesca Del Gado

About 15 years ago, Donatella Tomaiuoli realised that clients can easily learn to use fluency-enhancing techniques, but this is not enough. We often experience how difficult it is for clients to generalise what they learn during their treatment when they are in their everyday life, when there is no therapist with them.

Joseph Attanasio

So, are you saying that art-mediated therapy facilitates generalisation?

Francesca Del Gado

Yes, during the treatment, which includes art-mediated training such as theatre or dubbing, clients accept that they have to expose themselves to situations in which they have to match the demands of everyday conversation. Clients' perceived self-efficacy improves with facing a challenge, such as going on stage in front of a real audience and/or facing time pressure induced by dubbing in a recording studio. So, for example, when clients face an oral test at school, they think 'I was on stage for a theatre performance'or 'I was in a recording studio for dubbing', and 'if I did that, now I can do this'.

Ann Packman
How do you decide to move from speech therapy to the transfer activities, and then to the art-mediated training? Is it task mastery?

Francesca Del Gado
Yes, based on task mastery, we design a timetable for each profile. In our experience after 3 or 4 months of therapy, clients are ready for the next step. But steps overlap to some extent, so that skills from previous steps still feature in therapy but assume less importance with time.

Joseph Attanasio
This treatment is clearly driven by a view of what stuttering is. Could you just reiterate what stuttering is to you and how does it influence your treatment?

Francesca Del Gado
In our view the essence of treatment is never to forget that the client is first of all a person. Our multifactorial perspective recognises a genetic component, an attitude and an influence from the environment from client experiences. All of these are integrated into each client's story, and as such require an integrated treatment. We don't want to make clients think they will be perfectly fluent every time they speak. But we do want to give them the tools to enhance their fluency and the self-confidence to believe they are able to face every verbal situation of their lives, without avoidance reaction. We would like our clients to think, 'So I stutter, but this doesn't stop me from going to New York City' or 'putting up my hand in the classroom', and so on. We also use irony and humour to teach clients to joke with themselves. This is particularly important in children, as they soon learn a positive way to perceive and cope with their stuttering, which is useful for each of their social interactions and for their growth.

Sheena Reilly
Could you give us more details of the fluency-enhancing techniques you use?

Francesca Del Gado
We follow the techniques outlined by Professor Hugo Gregory, because he inspired us. We focus on what clients need most. For example, if a client talks very fast, we obviously work on slowing their speech.

Sheena Reilly
So, you use different techniques on different clients?

Francesca Del Gado
Yes, each client experiences different techniques based on self-modelling and fluency enhancing. We introduce them all, discuss the clients' points of view and then jointly decide the way to go with therapy.

Ann Packman

Our group thought that people from some cultures might not be willing to participate in theatrical aspects. Is theatre optional?

Francesca Del Gado

No, we can say we are not democratic with our clients. . . . But the length of our programme gives our clinicians time enough to build a sound relationship with clients, and obtain their trust and compliance. In fact, in the first period they do not often say 'Oh, theatre is great!' or 'Oh, dubbing is great! I can't wait to start'. Most of our clients say, 'Please, please, I want just individual therapy sessions'.

Each group activity is difficult for our clients; they don't feel comfortable with it. This is particularly true for theatre and dubbing, which are particularly challenging for clients who stutter. But as they go on with their treatment, they slowly change their mind about it. They realise that this training is important for them; that they are not alone in that activity, and there are clinicians there beside them during those activities.

Ann Packman

I think I would be reluctant.

Francesca Del Gado

Well, in such cases we say to our clients, 'Take your time to reconsider the matter'. And usually they do it. They manage their worries and their anxiety. And after the play they often say, 'I did it! I can do it again!' Just this year, we had to schedule a rerun of the final theatre performance because our clients asked us to. If we look back at our entire experience, we can say that in about 10 years perhaps only three clients avoided this experience.

Joseph Attanasio

Could you tell us the youngest client that you work with?

Francesca Del Gado

Children can start this programme from the age of seven. But we also have a programme for preschool children.

Sheena Reilly

Do you involve the parents of the children? Do they come along to the sessions?

Francesca Del Gado

We involve parents of children and adolescents' parents with counselling. We don't usually involve parents in the sessions with children, because they often simply tell their children to not stutter.

References

Andrews, G., & Cutler, J. (1974) Stuttering therapy: The relationship between changes in symptom level and attitudes. *Journal of Speech and Hearing Disorders, 38,* 312-319.

Campbell, J. H., & Hill, D. G. (1999) Systematic disfluency analysis. In: H. Gregory (Ed.), *Stuttering Therapy: A Workshop for Specialists* (pp. 51-76). Evanston, IL: Northwestern University & The Speech Foundation of America.

Cook, F., & Rustin, L. (1997) Commentary on the Lidcombe Programme of early stuttering intervention. *European Journal of Disorders in Communication, 32*, 250-258.

Craig, A. R., Franklin, J. A., & Andrews, G. (1984) A scale to measure locus of control of behaviour. *British Journal of Medical Psychology, 57*, 173-180.

Gregory, H. H. (2003) *Stuttering Therapy: Rationale and Procedures*. Boston, MA: Allyn & Bacon.

Hicks, R. (2005) The Iceberg Matrix of Stuttering. Paper presented at the ISAD 2005. Retrieved from http://www.mnsu.edu/comdis/isad8/papers/hicks8/hicks8.html

Schindler, O. (1980) *Handbook of Communication Disorders* (Vol. I.) Turin, Italy: Omega Edizioni.

Smith, A., & Kelly, E. (1997) Stuttering: a dynamic, multifactorial model. In: R. F. Curlee & G. M. Siegel (Eds.), *Nature and Treatment of Stuttering* (pp. 97-127). Boston: Allyn & Bacon.

Spielberger, C. D. (1983) *Manual for the State-Trait Anxiety Inventory*. Palo Alto, CA: Consulting Psychologists Press.

Starkweather, C. W., & Givens-Ackerman, C. R. (1997) *Stuttering*. Austin, TX: Pro-Ed.

Tomaiuoli, D. (2005) A theatrical approach to treating stuttering. *ASHA Leader*, 20-21.

Tomaiuoli, D., Castiglione, R., Del Gado, F., Falcone, P., Lucchini, E., Pasqua, E., & Spinetti, M. G. (2006) The use of movie and spot dubbing in stuttering treatment. In: J. Au-Yeung & M. M. Leahy (Eds.), *Research, Treatment, and Self-help in Fluency Disorders: New Horizons. Proceedings of the International Fluency Association's 5th World Congress* (pp. 130-135), Dublin, Ireland: International Fluency Association.

Tomaiuoli, D., Del Gado, F., Porchetti, G., Spinetti, M. G., & Falcone, P. (2009) Tales interpreted reading: a laboratory for children who stutter. Paper presented at the 6th World Congress on Fluency Disorders, Rio de Janeiro, Brazil.

Van Riper, C. (1982) *The Nature of Stuttering* (2nd ed.). Englewood Cliffs, NJ: Prentice Hall.

Yairi, E. (2007) Subtyping Stuttering I: a review. *Journal of Fluency Disorders, 32*, 165-196.

Yaruss, J. S., & Quesal, R. W. (2006) Overall Assessment of the Speaker's Experience of Stuttering (OASES). *Journal of Fluency Disorders, 31*, 90-115.

Yaruss, J. S., Coleman, C. E., & Quesal, R. W. (2006) Assessment of the Child's Experience of Stuttering (ACES). Poster presented at the Annual Convention of the American Speech-Language-Hearing Association, Miami, FL.

Woolf, G. (1967) The assessment of stuttering as struggle, avoidance, and expectancy. *British Journal of Disorders of Communication, 2*, 158-171.

Chapter 12

Self-Modelling for Chronic Stuttering

Angela Cream[1] and Sue O'Brian[2]

[1]*Osborne Park Hospital, Perth, Australia*
[2]*The University of Sydney, Sydney, Australia*

Overview

Self-modelling is a simple treatment for problem behaviour that involves observation of oneself without the problem behaviour. The purpose of self-modelling is to increase the rate of the desirable behaviour and decrease the rate of the undesirable behaviour. Most commonly, self-modelling incorporates a target video of ideal, error-free behaviour. In the case of stuttering, that model is stutter-free speech. Self-modelling treatment for stuttering involves first constructing a target video recording that is stutter free and then having the client watch the video repeatedly.

Ideally, target videos are short, typically less than 5 minutes duration. In order to provide variety of content or situations, more than one target video is usually constructed. The videos may involve a number of different speaking situations, for example, monologue (Cream et al., 2009), conversation (Bray and Kehle 1996, 1998; Webber et al., 2004) or telephone conversation (Cream et al., 2010). To attain a video that is stutter free, scripting, role-play or rehearsal can be used (Bray and Kehle, 1996, 1998). Another technique is to request the client to repeat all stuttered utterances while being video recorded until fluent speech is attained (Webber et al., 2004). If the client has been treated with speech restructuring (see Preface for a definition of this term) and is familiar with that technique, it can be used to attain stutter-free speech on the video recording (Cream et al., 2009, 2010). The resulting video is then edited to remove any stuttering that might remain. Editing can also produce scenarios to produce the illusion that the client is speaking to someone who was in fact not present during the recording. For example, the final video can appear as if a person in authority is asking the client questions to which the client responds.

The Science and Practice of Stuttering Treatment: A Symposium, First Edition. Edited by Suzana Jelčić Jakšić and Mark Onslow.
© 2012 John Wiley & Sons, Ltd. Published 2012 by John Wiley & Sons, Ltd.

Clients are provided with a copy of their target video, which they can view with a computer screen or television. Clients are instructed simply to speak as they do on the video. Viewing of videos by stuttering clients may occur once each day (Cream et al., 2009, 2010) or two to three times a week (Bray and Kehle, 1996, 1998).

Theoretical basis

Self-modelling is thought to provide a unique source of information that may contribute to behaviour change because (1) it influences judgements of self-efficacy through self-observation of the desirable behaviour, (2) information is provided about how best to perform skills through observational learning and (3) self-regulation as described by social cognitive theory is applied. These three theoretical characteristics of self-modelling are described in the following text.

Self-efficacy

Bandura (2001) described self-efficacy as the basis of human action. Levels of perceived self-efficacy affect motivation and the goals individuals set for themselves. According to social cognitive theory, self-efficacy reduces fear associated with anticipation, affects how much effort people will use and how long they will persist despite obstacles (Bandura, 2003). Perceived levels of self-efficacy are based on information that is integrated from a range of sources such as verbal persuasion and physical and psychological characteristics of the individual, for example, whether tired or in a depressed state of mind. A powerful source of information that can affect self-efficacy is thought to be mastery experiences of performing a behaviour successfully (Bandura, 1997; Schunk and Hanson, 1989).

Observational learning

Bandura (1997) and Schunk and Hanson (1989) also proposed that human behaviour is learned by observing models. Observational learning is more efficient than the trial and error approach of performing a behaviour followed by consequences, then trying again. Four processes determine whether a target behaviour is elicited following observational learning: (1) *attention*, meaning that observers need to attend to the model, (2) *retention* of the correct observed behaviour, (3) *reproduction* capacity to produce motoric features of the requisite behaviour and (4) *motivation* to attain the behaviour. Judgements derived from observational learning are mediated by an interaction between the characteristics of the observer, the nature of the model, as well as factors in the environment.

Self-regulation

The process of self-regulation, as described by social cognitive theory (Bandura, 1986), is thought to be inherent to self-modelling. Self-regulation refers to the capacity of humans to control their reactions or modify their environment rather than respond automatically to stimuli. A basic process of self-regulation is self-observation. Self-observation serves two functions in regulating behaviour. First, it provides the necessary information to set realistic performance standards and, second, it provides the necessary information to evaluate on-going changes in behaviour (Bandura, 1986). Self-modelling is a form of self-observation. Therapeutic use of self-modelling is thought to alter the client's self-observation about the problem behaviour, including the proportion of successes or failures to attain the desired behaviour.

Self-modelling also incorporates the judgmental process of self-regulation through the availability of comparisons. Internal standards of individuals affect the judgement about their actions. Internal standards can develop within individuals by using evaluative social reactions to their behaviour. During everyday life, people not only self-evaluate their reactions but also often voice the standards they are using to judge the adequateness or propriety of their behaviour. Therapeutic self-modelling demonstrations are more influential when standards are expressed in word as well as in action (Liebert et al., 1969).

In summary, self-modelling gives the observer the opportunity to reflect on the consequences of their own behaviour rather than relying on learning from others. This is in contrast to observational learning where others are the models. Thus self-observation helps a client to differentiate the kinds of responses that lead to particular consequences. In this way, self-observation can be considered to play a mediation role in the regulation of behaviour (Bandura, 1977).

Demonstrated value

There are now sufficient clinical trials of this treatment to warrant its consideration as an adjunct to standard methods for stuttering control. Bray and Kehle (1996, 1998) reported two laboratory experiments with self-modelling, both of which were multiple baseline across subjects designs. The participants watched stutter-free target videos in the clinic with an investigator present approximately once a week for a period of 5-6 weeks. These studies demonstrated that stuttering was responsive to self-modelling, results were durable over time and that the participants were satisfied with the treatment.

The Bray and Kehle (1996) report involved three adolescents aged 13-17 years, all of whom had previously learnt a speech restructuring technique for stuttering control. Their mean percentage of syllables stuttered (%SS) during conversational speech pre-treatment was 36, 40 and 18 for Participants 1, 2 and 3, respectively. Stuttering reduced considerably at the end of the intervention period to 5, 9 and 4 %SS, respectively. The Bray and Kehle

(1998) study replicated those findings with four younger participants aged 8-13 years, two of whom had previous speech restructuring treatment. The mean percentage of stuttered words for Participants 1-4 was 7.7, 5.9, 9.1 and 8.0, respectively, which reduced to 4.8, 2.6, 4.2 and 0.2, respectively, at post-treatment. Stuttering reduced still further at follow-up for 3 of the 4 participants; 2.6, 1.5, 3.2 and 0.3 percent stuttered words.

Bray and Kehle (2001) reported a long-term follow-up of these participants 2 and 4 years later. Four of the seven participants retained below 4 %SS. One participant maintained his initial stuttering reduction while the last two increased their stuttering rates. Bray and Kehle (1998) suggested that self-modelling may have been of the most value to the participants with variable stuttering across situations. They reported that self-modelling appeared to reduce levels of stuttering during situations that had been problematic for participants. A limitation of the three Bray and Kehle (1996, 1998, 2001) reports was that speech samples were collected in the presence of the investigator, hence raising the possibility of bias because of discriminated learning of stuttering control. Further, individual participants in the follow-up study cannot be identified.

Webber et al. (2004) studied self-modelling in a carefully controlled laboratory study to determine its effects on stuttering. Participants were two men aged 22 and 29 years and one adolescent boy aged 17 years. An important feature of this study was that none of the participants had a history of speech restructuring treatment. The target self-modelling videos for the experiment were constructed by editing an interview with an off-camera clinician. Each participant was studied with a single subject additive-design experiment consisting of A, B and B+C Phases. In each phase participants spoke in monologue for 3-minute trials.

Subsequent to the baseline A Phase, participants watched their target videos prior to each speaking period during a B Phase. In the B+C Phase, participants continued to watch the video prior to each speaking period but were also instructed to talk as they had on the video. Two participants reduced stuttering in both the B and B+C conditions, however an independent rater verified findings for only one of these participants. Although self-modelling in the laboratory did show stimulus control for one participant, generally the results were not as pronounced as with the Bray and Kehle studies (1996, 1998).

The findings by Webber et al. (2004) indicated that self-modelling alone may not be sufficient to reduce chronic stuttering. Self-observation of stutter-free speech may increase levels of self-efficacy, however, the model alone may not provide sufficient information on how to produce stutter-free speech. Theoretically, observers need the physical ability to *reproduce* the stutter-free speech demonstrated in the self-modelling video. Webber and colleagues noted that participants in the Bray and Kehle (1996) study had all had speech restructuring treatment, which may have contributed to the results, but this was not the case for their study.

Cream et al. (2009) noted the potential for self-modelling to assist clients with speech restructuring stuttering control. Participants in their study were

10 adults who had relapsed following speech restructuring treatment. There was a mean time since treatment of 25 years. Target videos were constructed from a 1-hour videotaped speaking session with a clinician, during which pe-riod they were encouraged to use their speech pattern to control stuttering on the target videos. These videos were given to participants with instructions to watch the video twice a day for a period of 1 month. Assessments occurred before and immediately following the 1-month self-modelling intervention pe-riod. The primary outcome measure was %SS based on beyond-clinic conver-sational samples. The secondary outcome measures were participant severity measures based on a 9-point severity rating scale where 1 = *no stuttering*, 2 = *very mild stuttering* and 9 = *extremely severe stuttering*; and speech naturalness, where 1 = *extremely natural-sounding speech* and 9 = *extremely unnatural-sounding speech* (Martin et al., 1984). Severity measures were col-lected for a range of situations nominated by participants as representing typical, easy and difficult situations. The group mean %SS pre-treatment was 7.7 and 2.3 post-treatment, a difference of 5.4 %SS (95% CI = 1.89–8.89 %SS, $t(9) = 3.49$, $p < 0.0001$). This was a very large effect size of 1.1 (Cohen's *d*; (mean 1 – mean 2)/pooled standard deviation). The group mean severity rating pre-intervention was 4.4 and 3.1 post-intervention; a difference of 1.7 (95% CI = 1.35–2.13, $t(9) = 10.15$, $p < 0.0001$). This was a very large effect size of 1.4 (Cohen's *d*; (mean 1 – mean 2)/pooled standard deviation). Participant severity ratings reduced for all participants across a range of speaking situa-tions, including those they found most difficult. The mean speech naturalness scores of 3.8 pre-intervention and 3.9 post-intervention were unchanged. A limitation of this study was the lack of follow-up data. However, the findings supported the notion that self-modelling is a viable procedure for adults who stutter when combined with speech restructuring treatment.

Using the Onslow et al. (2008) definition of a clinical trial,[1] there has been only one trial of self-modelling. This was the Cream et al. (2010) trial of the procedure as an adjunct to speech restructuring. Participants were 89 ado-lescents and adults. At the end of a 5-day Instatement Phase of speech re-structuring treatment, participants were randomly assigned to two trial arms: standard maintenance or standard maintenance plus self-modelling. Partici-pants in the self-modelling group were requested to view stutter-free videos of themselves each day for 1 month.

The primary outcome measure was %SS. Secondary outcome measures in-cluded self-reported stuttering severity, a Subjective Units of Distress Scale score (Wolpe, 1958), levels of satisfaction with fluency and quality of life mea-sured with the Overall Assessment of the Speaker's Experience of Stuttering (OASES) for adults (Yaruss and Quesal, 2006) and adolescents (Yaruss et al., 2010). The major finding from this study at 6 months post-treatment was that there was no significant difference between groups for %SS, however, there were significant differences in self-report measures between the groups. For the self-modelling group, self-rated worst stuttering severity was 0.5 scale

---

[1] A prospective attempt to determine the efficacy of an entire treatment based on at least 3 months follow-up observations of speech beyond the clinic (Onslow et al., 2008).

values lower, or 10% better than for the control group (95% CI = -1.6 to -0.2, p = 0.012). Satisfaction with fluency was 20% better than the control group. The difference was 0.8 scale values (95% CI = -1.7 to 0.0, p = 0.043). The total impact of stuttering on quality of life as measured by the OASES/ Assessment of the Child's Experience of Stuttering (ACES) was less for the self-modelling group, which rated mild-moderately impaired while the control group was moderately impaired (95% CI = -10 to -0.6, p = 0.027). The results of this trial are overviewed in Figure 12.1.

Both studies that investigated the use of self-modelling in conjunction with speech restructuring (Cream et al., 2009, 2010) reported positive changes in self-reported severity ratings. Taken together, they therefore provide support for the notion that self-modelling may contribute to the generalisation of treatment effects; particularly considering that one of them warrants interpretation as a clinical trial. Overall satisfaction with fluency and reduced impact of stuttering may be related to a change in perceived self-efficacy.

A limitation of all the evidence presented here is that self-efficacy is theoretically considered to be underpinning self-modelling treatment, however, none of the studies reviewed have measured it. In summary, although the objective measures do not give a consistently positive result, the self-report measures demonstrate some value of self-modelling for chronic stuttering.

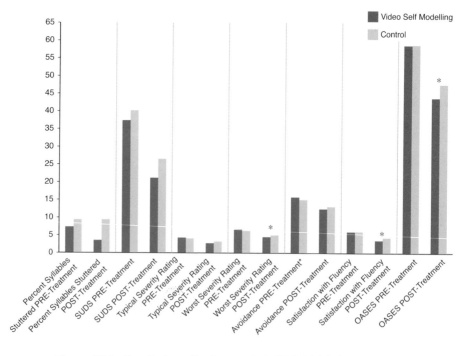

Figure 12.1 Results from the Cream et al. (2010) trial at pre-treatment and at 6 months post-randomisation (OASES = quality of life measured with the OASES for adults and adolescents; * = p < 0.05).

The evidence from these six studies shows that there is great potential for self-modelling as an adjunct to speech restructuring treatment for chronic stuttering.

Advantages and disadvantages

Advantages

Self-modelling for chronic stuttering is a simple and cost efficient treatment that has potential to reduce stuttered speech, particularly following speech restructuring treatment. Self-report measures indicate it has potential to promote both generalisation and maintenance of speech outcomes. It appears that all clinicians need to do to potentially bring these benefits to clients is to supplement their treatments with a self-modelling video recording. There are striking cost efficiencies to such a procedure. Arguably the literature reviewed suggests that self-modelling may be particularly applicable to the problem of post-treatment relapse. If the findings of Cream et al. (2009) can be replicated, it is conceivable that all clients could finish their treatments armed with a self-modelling video, and it could be used to restore stuttering control as needed. Perhaps the problem of post-treatment relapse may be considerably diminished if clients were to regularly review their self-modelling recording.

Disadvantages

The disadvantage of self-modelling is that clients need to have the ability to produce reasonable amounts of stutter-free speech for their self-modelling recording. Beyond that practicality, based on the evidence presented here, self-modelling appears to be efficacious for stuttering clients who have already learned a speech restructuring technique to control stuttered speech. At least judging from the Webber et al. (2004) results, those who have never learned any technique for stuttering control do not respond as favourably as those who have received some such treatment. It is also the case that the clinical trials reported here show a modest effect size. If further clinical trials affirm that indeed such an effect size is all that is realistically attainable with self-modelling, then, considering that such effects can be attained without any clinical cost, then they would be worth having nonetheless.

Conclusions and future directions

There is considerable potential for self-modelling as an adjunct treatment for stuttering. Nonetheless, there are many targets for further investigation. There are three research directions from now that would guide clinical practice. The first relates to the theory that underpins self-modelling. Can the self-efficacy changes that relate to self-modelling be measured? At present it is assumed, rather than proven, that the benefits of the procedure during stuttering treatment are related to such changes in self-efficacy. If it can be shown that this is the case, then clinicians could focus more specifically on self-efficacy during self-modelling as an adjunct treatment to stuttering. Second, and most fundamentally, further clinical trials research is needed to verify the potential benefits of the procedure. Using a liberal definition of a clinical trial, only one has been reported. Independent replication of clinical trials results is essential to bolster clinician confidence in that result. Finally, it seems to be a general rule of stuttering treatment that interventions are more efficacious for younger participants, but that does not appear to be the case with self-modelling. That certainly requires continued research.

It has been demonstrated that even a brief delay between performance and observation reduces the instructive value of the self-modelling (Carroll & Bandura, 1985; Fireman, 1996). Performance is enhanced, however, when video feedback is provided simultaneously with a behaviour that could otherwise not be observed by the person (Carroll & Bandura, 1982). For example, simultaneous self-modelling displays presented in a mirror rather than by video have been used in conjunction with negative practice to reduce the frequency of facial tics (Frederick, 1971). An early recommendation by Van Riper (1973) was that those who stutter should read in front of a mirror. Subsequent investigations of this idea (Hudock et al., 2011; Snyder et al., 2009) suggested some merit in it, and a programme of research at the Australian Stuttering Research Centre has begun to explore it further.

Our progress to date is an experiment with ten stuttering clients, five of whom had previously learnt a speech restructuring technique to control stuttering and five of whom had had no previous treatment. A time series single subject ABA design was used. The A_1 phase involved speaking in monologue for 3-minute trials, the B phase involved speaking in monologue for 3-minute trials while looking into a mirror and the A_2 phase was a repeat A_1 phase. Eight participants completed the experiment and for seven of these, no effect on stuttering from mirror self-modelling was evident. However, stuttering did reduce for one participant who had previously learnt a speech restructuring technique to control stuttering. Results for this participant are presented in Figure 12.2. We are not sure yet what to make of this modest finding, but there is some possibility that further research will show that for some clients who experience post-treatment relapse, mirror self-modelling may be a useful technique.

Discussion

Joseph Attanasio

One question we had is why does it work? You mentioned Bandura's theorising. We were wondering, have Bandura's theories of self-modelling been empirically supported? Can we be sure that it works because of those theoretical positions?

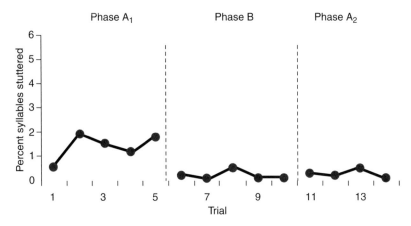

Figure 12.2 Results for one of the successful participants from our preliminary investigation of mirror self-modelling.

Angela Cream

I suppose teasing out and testing why a treatment works often comes late in its development. The short answer to your question is that the underpinning theory has certainly not been scrutinised empirically. But the underpinning theory of self-modelling is accepted for all applications of self-modelling beyond stuttering management.

Sheena Reilly

I want to ask you about whether you think this is a suitable approach for all types of personalities. Are there contraindications for using it for some clients? Would there be clinical differences in its value for clients with different types of learning styles, for example?

Angela Cream

Bandura (1986) considered that the characteristics of an individual affect whether or not an observed behaviour will be imitated. We all have internal standards for our performance based on previous experience and individual ways of interpreting information. For example, if a person's self-expectation is higher than what is achieved, even though suitable, the self-focus may be on being unsuccessful. One of the benefits of self-modelling is that it helps to moderate this internal standard. Schunk and Hanson (1989) reported on some differences in responses. Learning styles is an interesting suggestion for a research direction. So far as I am aware, it has not been studied with self-modelling and stuttering.

Sheena Reilly

Our group wondered how compliant participants were during these studies. Do you know how they felt about using the self-modelling technique?

Angela Cream

In the first study I mentioned (Cream et al., 2009), clients were asked to watch a 5-minute video twice a day. All participants complied according to their log except one, who had around 80% compliance. However, in the randomised control trial the compliance was not as favourable (Cream et al., 2010). We don't know the reason for that; participants only had to watch the video once a day and the video was shorter than the previous trial at only $3\frac{1}{2}$ minutes. However, perhaps it had something to do with the self-modelling target video being not as important to them at the time, just after a clinical trial, as it was with the former study when relapse had occurred. According to its underpinning theory, for self-modelling to work, you need to (1) have attention to the model, (2) remember the model, (3) be able to reproduce the technique and also (4) be motivated. Now, at the end of a speech restructuring treatment programme when they are still in maintenance, clients may not have had the motivation to watch themselves being stutter free on a video because they were free of stuttering most of the time. And consequently they may not have needed or wanted to attend to the video. But then again, there was really was no reason for them to watch it every day. In the Bray and Kehle (1996, 1998) studies, the videos were watched only six times in total to attain an effect. In the randomised control trial (Cream et al., 2010), even though there was not daily compliance by all participants, there was still a significant effect. Perhaps people are able to self-select when they watch themselves. Certainly, in the wider self-modelling literature, it is routinely acknowledged that very few viewings are needed to effect a change.

Joseph Attanasio
Our group suggests an iPod app for clients to use during everyday situations. But you have to share the profits.

Angela Cream
Indeed, some clients said after treatment that they may watch their target video if they know that they are going into a situation in which they don't want to stutter. So that is a fine idea.

Joseph Attanasio
Does the self-modelling recording need to be video or is audio only satisfactory?

Angela Cream
No, not at all. The trials I have been involved with used target videos, so that is why I mentioned videos a lot. The literature indicates that audio only is fine. But certainly it is clinically intuitive to use a video with stuttering.

Sheena Reilly
The Bray and Kehle participants were quite young. Do you think this would work with even younger children, say 5-7 years old?

Angela Cream
The youngest participant in those studies was 8 years old. Outside the stuttering literature, there is evidence for positive results from self-modelling when used with children who are 5 years old, for example, see Buggey, 2005.

Theoretically self-modelling could work if participants had the four pre-requisites outlined earlier of attention, retention, ability to reproduce the behaviour and motivation. However, Clarke et al. (1993) suggested younger children may not have this capacity, and self-modelling may not be sufficient to effect change with younger children, aged 3–5 years.

Ann Packman

Do you see this as a stand-alone treatment or do you think it is best as an adjunct?

Angela Cream

Of course, that is an empirical question, but in theory it could be a stand-alone intervention for those who have the motor capacity to control stuttering. The Cream et al. (2009) trial showed that. Perhaps that ultimately will be shown to be its most powerful use, to redress relapse problems. One reason I was led a moment ago to guess that it does not produce optimal results with younger children is that they just don't have that motor capacity. It needs to be learned through treatment later during life.

Ann Packman

Our group discussed whether looking at the same video is boring for clients.

Angela Cream

It probably is boring for some people, but on the up side, the benefits from self-modelling appear to be attainable with just minimal viewing. A questionnaire in the Cream et al. (2010) study at the end of the 28 days viewing time asked participants what the worst thing about self-modelling was. Eight percent responded that it was boring. After 5 months, the participants who were not watching the DVD were asked the reason and 6% reported feeling sick of it.

References

Bandura, A. (1977) Self-efficacy: toward a unifying theory of behavior change. *Psychological Review, 84*, 191–215.

Bandura, A. (1986) *Social Foundations of Thought and Action: A Social Cognitive Theory*. Englewood Cliffs, NJ: Prentice-Hall.

Bandura, A. (1997) *Self-efficacy: The Exercise of Control*. New York: Freeman.

Bandura, A. (2001) Social cognitive theory: an agentic perspective. *Annual Review of Psychology, 52*, 1–26.

Bandura, A. (2003) Role of affective self-regulatory efficacy in diverse spheres of psychosocial functioning. *Child Development, 74*, 769–782.

Bray, M. A., & Kehle, T. J. (1996) Self-modeling as an intervention for stuttering. *School Psychology Review, 25*, 358–369.

Bray, M. A., & Kehle, T. J. (1998) Self-modeling as an intervention for stuttering. *School Psychology Review, 27*, 587–598.

Bray, M. A., & Kehle, T. J. (2001) Long-term follow-up of self-modeling as an intervention for stuttering. *School Psychology Review, 30*, 135–141.

Buggey, T. (2005) Video self-modeling applications with students with autism spectrum disorder in a small private school setting. *Focus on Autism and Other Developmental Disabilities, 20*, 52–53.

Carroll, W. R., & Bandura, A. (1982) The role of visual monitoring in observational learning of action patterns: making the unobservable observable. *Journal of Motor Behavior, 14,* 153-167.

Carroll, W. R., & Bandura, A. (1985) Role of timing of visual monitoring and motor rehearsal in observational learning of action patterns. *Journal of Motor Behavior, 17*(3), 269-281.

Clarke, E., Beck, D., Sloane, H., Jenson, W., Bowen, J., Goldsmith, D, & Kehle, T. (1993) Self-modeling with pre-schoolers: is it different? *School Psychology International, 14,* 83-89.

Cream, A., O'Brian, S., Onslow, M., Packman, A., & Menzies, R. (2009) Self-modelling as a relapse intervention following speech-restructuring treatment for stuttering. *International Journal of Language and Communication Disorders, 44,* 587-599.

Cream, A., O'Brian, S., Jones, M., Block, S., Harrison, E., Lincoln, M., & Onslow, M. (2010) Randomized controlled trial of video self-modeling following speech restructuring treatment for stuttering. *Journal of Speech, Language, and Hearing Research, 53,* 1-11.

Fireman, G. (1996) Developing a plan for problem solving: a representational shift. *Cognitive Development, 11,* 107-122.

Frederick, C. (1971) Treatment of a tic by a systematic desensitization and massed response evocation. *Journal of Behavioral Therapy and Experimental Psychiatry, 2,* 281-283.

Hudock, D., Dayalu, V., Saltuklaroglu, T., Stuart, A., Zhang, J., & Kalinowski, J. (2011) Stuttering inhibition via visual feedback at normal and fast speech rates. *International Journal of Language and Communication Disorders, 46*(2), 169-178.

Liebert, R. M., Hanratty, M., & Hill, J. H. (1969) Effects of rule structure and training method on the adoption of a self-imposed standard. *Child Development, 40,* 93-101.

Martin, R. R., Haroldson, S. K., & Triden, K. A. (1984) Stuttering and speech naturalness. *Journal of Speech and Hearing Disorders, 49,* 53-58.

Onslow, M., Jones, M., O'Brian, S., Menzies, R., & Packman, A. (2008) Defining, identifying, and evaluating clinical trials of stuttering treatments: a tutorial for clinicians. *American Journal of Speech Language Pathology, 17,* 401-415.

Schunk, D. H., & Hanson, A. R. (1989) Self-modeling and children's cognitive skill learning. *Journal of Educational Psychology, 81,* 155-163.

Snyder, G., Hough, M., Blanchet, P., Ivy, L., & Waddell, D. (2009) The effects of self-generated synchronous and asynchronous visual speech feedback on overt stuttering frequency. *Journal of Communication Disorders, 42*(3), 235-244.

Van Riper, C. (1973) The Treatment of Stuttering. Englewood Cliffs, NJ: Prentice-Hall.

Webber, M. J., Packman, A., & Onslow, M. (2004) Effects of self-modelling on stuttering. *International Journal of Language and Communication Disorders, 39,* 509-522.

Wolpe, J. (1958) *Psychotherapy by Reciprocal Inhibition.* Stanford, CA: Stanford University Press.

Yaruss, J. S., & Quesal, R. W. (2006) Overall assessment of the speaker's experience of stuttering (OASES): documenting multiple outcomes in stuttering treatment. *Journal of Fluency Disorders, 31,* 90-115.

Yaruss, J. S., Quesal, R. W., & Coleman, C. (2010) *OASES:Overall Assessment of the Speaker's Experience of Stuttering: Ages 13-17.* Bloomington, MN: Pearson Assessments.

Chapter 13

Multifactorial Treatment for Preschool Children

Mirjana Lasan

Logopedski Centar, Zagreb, Croatia

Overview

In a more real sense than other early interventions, multifactorial treatments are family-based treatments. They are indirect treatments, which attempt to ameliorate a child's stuttering by changing linguistic and communication behaviours of other family members, and by other modifications to the child's living environment.

Data-based reports of the multifactorial style of treatment suggest that current prominent models worldwide are Parent Child Interaction (PCI) therapy (The Michael Palin Centre, London) and Family Focused Treatment (Stuttering Centre of West Pennsylvania, United States). The treatments are designed for children between 2 and 6 years of age. Both versions include parent-focused strategies as well as child-focused strategies, with the former being addressed first.

In the PCI approach the initial assessment, which consists of a child assessment and parent consultation, is followed by six sessions, 1 hour long, of clinic-based therapy, 6 weeks of home-based therapy and regular review sessions for up to 1 year post-treatment. Depending on factors thought to have an impact on a particular child's stuttering, several parent-focused strategies are used. Parents implement other strategies such as helping children manage emotions about stuttering and confidence building. Direct child speech strategies such as using easy onsets, rate reduction or pausing are administered only if children continue to stutter after the implementation of parent-focused strategies

During the first PCI session Special Time is arranged. Special Time is a 5-minute play period that each parent has with the stuttering child, 3-5 times each week. Within home-based therapy, parents continue with Special Time and the aim is for parents to generalise skills learned in the clinic into the

The Science and Practice of Stuttering Treatment: A Symposium, First Edition. Edited by Suzana Jelčić Jakšić and Mark Onslow.

home environment. Each child's progress is reviewed at 3 weeks, 3 months, 6 months and 12 months post-clinic.

The parent-child training programme of Family Focused Treatment consists of 6-9 sessions, 45 minutes long, once per week. It comprises three components: (1) education and counselling about communication and stuttering (2-4 sessions), (2) communication modification training (3 sessions) and (3) review and reassessment (1-2 sessions) in which parents evaluate their use of the treatment strategies.

Although the aim of both treatments is to reduce stuttering, their descriptions contain no overt statement that no stuttering or almost no stuttering is part of their treatment goals (Millard et al., 2008, 2009; Yaruss et al., 2006). The treatments focus instead on counselling and educating parents about stuttering and assisting them to deal with their children's stuttering through modifying parent communication behaviours, along with linguistic and environmental factors. Both treatments explain that by manipulating these factors children may achieve more fluent speech.

Theoretical basis

The commonalities of these treatment styles suggest that they are derived from the thinking underlying multifactorial theory (for an overview see Packman and Attanasio, 2004). There are many factors posited by multifactorial theory to trigger and sustain stuttering during the preschool years. Those multiple factors combine and do so in a unique fashion for every child, with no single factor responsible for any case of stuttering. Arguably, most of the modern structure of these therapies was prompted by the thinking underlying the Demands and Capacities model (Starkweather, 1987). This model proposes that stuttering occurs because of an imbalance between demands for fluency and a child's capacity to be fluent. The main assumption of that model is that stuttering is most likely to occur when demands for fluency from the child's social environment exceed the child's cognitive, linguistic, motor or emotional capacities for fluent speech. The modifiable nature of the many demands for fluency is shown in Figure 13.1.

The PCI approach rests on the research interpretation that physiological and linguistic factors may be significant in the onset and development of stuttering and that their interaction with emotional and environmental aspects contributes to the severity and persistence of the disorder (Kelman et al., 2005). The Yaruss et al. (2006) description of Family Focused Treatment describes children's capacity for fluent speech as a bucket of water. The analogy shows that certain factors add water to the bucket and if the child's bucket becomes too full, the water spills out and the child stutters. Factors causing this could include (1) aspects of the child's overall development, such as perfectionism, high degree of sensitivity and genetic predisposition to stutter; (2) interpersonal stressors such as major changes or traumatic events in the child's life, marital conflicts, unrealistic developmental demands being placed

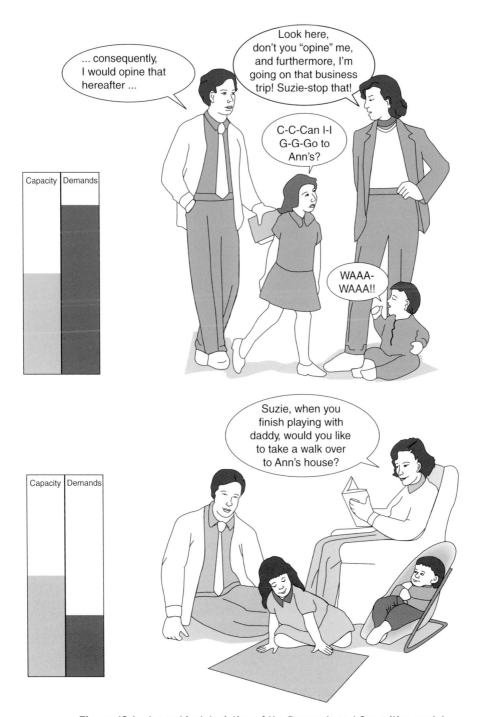

Figure 13.1 A graphical depiction of the Demands and Capacities model (Guitar, 2006). Used with permission.

on the child or fast-paced lifestyle and (3) communicative stressors that can increase the child's sense of time pressure, such as listener negative response to stuttering, frequent interruptions, rapid rate of conversation and competition for talking time. This analogy is supplemented with the explanation that the greater the child's intrinsic motor and linguistic skill, the greater the bucket size.

Because children differ in the combination of factors that may influence the onset and persistence of stuttering (Rustin et al., 1996), both treatments emphasise the necessity for an individual approach. Also, as mentioned previously, both approaches contend that manipulating aspects of the environment increases the likelihood that the child will be able to speak more fluently. So, the parent-focused aspects of both treatments seek to recognise and change those behaviours that may influence the child's stuttering. These may include reducing parent speech rate, increasing response time latency, reducing linguistic complexity, commenting rather than asking questions and following the child's lead in play.

Both treatments incorporate reduced parent speech rate, with associated slower conversational turn-taking patterns. Meyers and Freeman (1985) reported that parents of stuttering children spoke faster than control mothers to stuttering and control preschoolers. Zebrowski et al. (1996) reported some effect on stuttering when parents reduced speech rate, but the effect was by no means consistent. Yaruss and Conture (1995) similarly reported that the relation between parent speech rate and stuttering of preschoolers was not straightforward. In short, there is some evidence that reduced speech rate and altering turn-taking patterns will facilitate fluency, but their mechanisms are poorly understood (Bernstein Ratner, 2004). By consciously slowing speech rate, parents also change behaviours such as making longer turn-taking latencies (Bernstein Ratner, 1992), which, in turn, have been linked to reductions in stuttering frequency (Newman and Smit, 1989).

Demonstrated value

Yaruss et al. (2006) conducted a file audit of the Family Focused Treatment and evaluated preschoolers stuttering before and after the treatment and at follow-up, and gave parents a questionnaire. For the 17 children involved, there were significant reductions in the children's stuttering frequency in the clinical setting after the treatment. The mean stuttering frequency before treatment, in terms of stutters per 100 words, was 16.4% (SD = 6.6%) and at post-treatment was 3.2% (SD = 2.0%). Results of parents' ratings of treatment helpfulness and satisfaction showed that most parents were pleased with the components of the parent–child training programme and judged parent education about stuttering to be the most valuable. Their ratings of the children's speech showed that children spoke significantly more fluently following treatment at home and in new speaking situations.

Treatment outcomes and long-term follow-up indicate that 11 of the 17 children (64.7%) exhibited sufficient improvements in stuttering following the parent-child training programme and were dismissed from stuttering therapy entirely. Another six children (35%) continued to stutter and were enrolled in child-focused treatment, after which they were dismissed from treatment.

Millard et al. (2008) reported data from six young children who stutter who were involved in PCI. Stuttering severity was based on stuttering rate measured with percent syllables stuttered (%SS), duration of three longest stutters and the degree of tension and secondary behaviour present. This generated a score on a scale from 0 (normal speech) to 7 (very severe stuttering) (Yairi and Ambrose, 1992). The results of this Phase I clinical trial show that four of six children significantly reduced the frequency of their stuttering. Three of those four reduced stuttering severity to zero. One child reduced stuttering only with his father and continued with the therapy while the remaining child made significant progress when a direct approach was introduced.

Another study (Millard et al., 2009) investigating the efficacy of PCI showed results for 10 children. The study involved a Baseline Phase, followed by 6 weeks of clinic-based therapy and then 6 weeks of home-based therapy, then a Follow-up Phase. Six of the ten children received therapy and the other four did not. Millard et al. (2009) did not present the customary absolute measures of stuttering frequency, but analysed them with a cusum analysis. Results showed that there was a reduction in the trend of stuttering for four of the six children who received therapy. Three of four children remaining on the waiting list showed no systematic changes in stuttering, and the remaining one demonstrated a significant reduction, which the authors explained as spontaneous recovery. Parent ratings of the impact of stuttering on themselves and their confidence in managing the stuttering indicated improvements after the treatment.

Franken et al. (2005) compared the 12 weeks of Lidcombe Program (LP) treatment with 12 weeks of a treatment based on the Demands and Capacities model. The latter treatment was described as involving traditional Demands and Capacities components as needed, such as calming the household, modelling normal disfluencies and speaking to children with short, simple sentences. Three core components were presented to each family: (1) a special talking time each day dedicated exclusively to the child and designed to build self-confidence about speaking, (2) parent instruction to reduce speech rate and pause between utterances and (3) parent instruction not to overtly require any form of speech performance from children. Thirty children were randomly allocated to each of the therapies. Stuttering frequency and severity ratings were obtained immediately before and after 12 weeks of treatment. Both groups showed similar and significant reductions of stuttering frequency in %SS from 7.2% to 3.7% for the LP and from 7.9% to 3.1% for the Demands and Capacities model treatment. Similar results occurred as well for stuttering severity rated by parents: from 5.0 to 2.3 for the LP and from 4.8 to 2.1 for the Demands and Capacities model therapy. Overall, no differences between groups were found and parents rated both treatments favourably.

It is difficult to interpret the Franken et al. (2005) report because only portions of the treatments were presented and a no-treatment control group was not used to determine whether there was in fact any treatment effect or natural recovery was observed for the two experimental groups. Similar caveats apply to the results of the Yaruss et al. 2006 report and the two Phase I non-randomised clinical trials (Millard et al., 2008, 2009). Nonetheless, there is a strong suggestion that therapies based on the multifactorial model of early stuttering provide some stuttering reduction and parent understanding of their children's stuttering, and their capacity to cope with it will improve with counselling

Advantages and disadvantages

Advantages

The strength of the treatment is linked to the value of its guiding theory. Since the multifactorial model is about what triggers stuttering during childhood speech development, the model is not threatened by recent advances in the understanding of the more distant physiological causes of stuttering. At the beginning of both treatments, parents are taught about the multifactorial nature of stuttering and that those factors vary from one child to another, from one situation to another and from one time to another. This way parents learn that there is no single cause of stuttering and that they are not to blame for their child's stuttering. Hence, each child's stuttering treatment is individualised. They also learn that there are factors which are not under their control, such as genetic and temperament factors, and factors that can be modified, such as negative responses to stuttering, rapid rate of speech and coping with children who are sensitive about stuttering. This way parents become less anxious and by being active participants in treatment, parents become competent in dealing with their child's stuttering and helping the child to develop more effective communication skills and attitudes. The child, therefore, feels supported by parents. Also, as Kelman et al. (2005) suggest, the PCI approach – and indeed any approach based on a multifactorial model – can be implemented with very young children who still do not have well-developed attention and listening skills, or cognitive or meta-linguistic skills. Arguably, direct therapy would not be indicated for such children. The approach encourages parents to acknowledge their child's stuttering, but because the focus of the initial stages is not on the child's speech this could be useful for sensitive children who may interpret direct therapy as stuttering behaviour not being acceptable.

Disadvantages

Indirect approaches to early stuttering intervention, such as those overviewed here, could be criticised for an unproven theoretical basis and limited evidence of efficacy. Additionally, it is possible that such approaches may elicit parental blame about the disorder (Kelman et al., 2005). Obviously, this could have a negative impact on parents. Additionally, not all families are willing or able to participate in family-based approaches. As with some other family-based approaches it is hard to determine which components of the treatment contribute to any of its demonstrated efficacy and which are irrelevant. Another disadvantage is that the treatment is not overtly designed to remove children's stuttering, only to improve it.

All that being said, however, any proposed early intervention is likely to be controversial, and this is no exception. So, to what extent is a multifactorial model acceptable? To what extent does it fulfil the requirements of a successful theory: testability, heuristic value and explanatory power as outlined by Packman and Attanasio (2004)? Perhaps that is not for me to posit but to invite later discussion about.

Conclusions and future directions

The results of the Yaruss et al. (2006) preliminary study, the Franken et al. (2005) experiment, and the two Phase I clinical trials by Millard et al. (2008, 2009), have shown that some children involved in the PCI programme achieve stuttering reductions. Additionally, such interventions clearly increase parent knowledge and understanding of their child's stuttering, which helps them to deal with it. It is not clear at present, though, whether that intervention is better ultimately than no intervention. For some children, a more direct approach clearly is needed. This raises the question of the large-scale research that would eventually be needed to determine subgroups of children who are likely to benefit from such direct intervention rather than experiencing a delay in receiving it.

As with any treatment for early stuttering, the future of the treatments overviewed here, based on a multifactorial model of early stuttering, depends on research about that model itself and whether it can be successfully applied to early stuttering intervention. So, although the results of the preliminary clinical trials research show overall positive results, that is only the beginning. Franken et al. (2005) raised the prospect that parent involvement and time spent with children might be the critical elements of these indirect styles of treatment. That of course applies to any early stuttering intervention and beckons for experimental investigation. PCI has changed since it was initially developed. There is no reason to believe that treatment will continue to change and evolve over time in light of research and clinical experience. The same is true of Family Focused Treatment. Indeed, the authors of the report about that treatment reviewed here conclude that with further research such a treatment 'may ultimately take its place alongside other empirically validated approaches for helping young children who stutter develop and maintain normally fluent speech' (Yaruss et al., 2006, p. 130). Perhaps it is the most heartening feature of the work described here that the other two research groups involved (Franken et al., 2005; Millard et al., 2008, 2009) projected further empirical development of the treatments concerned.

Discussion[1]

Sheena Reilly

The first thing is to clarify that the main goal of the programme is to change the parents' behaviour and if so, we had a number of questions about how you actually measure that. How do you know that you've actually changed the parent behaviour?

Mirjana Lasan

This clinical approach would not necessarily be my first choice. You are correct that the emphasis is on changing parent behaviour and their communication with children. Unlike child stuttering severity, that is not so easy to measure. What you are raising is treatment fidelity. All treatments require parents to do certain things outside the clinic and it is a difficult matter to determine whether they actually do them.

Joseph Attanasio

Your presentation resonated with many in my group because of the focus on the child and not on the stuttering, and not using techniques to modify stuttering but to increase the opportunity for fluency. That led though to an inevitable comparison to the LP. The LP and the approaches you describe make use of parent interaction with children, albeit different kinds of interaction and for different purposes. Do you think that parent interaction with children could be important as a supportive variable with either programme?

Mirjana Lasan

Yes, of course that is a possibility.

Joseph Attanasio

Perhaps for future clinical trials we need a control condition where parents are just interacting with their children in a positive way. So the LP and, say, PCI therapy could be compared to a control condition in a randomised trial. The control condition could just involve positive parent attention to speech.

Dave Rowley

Of course that scientifically makes sense. But I can't really see how the two treatments could be combined in a clinical trial, because they have different primary outcomes. It seems to be a logical impossibility. The primary outcome for the LP is no stuttering or extremely mild stuttering, but that is not the case for PCI therapy, or any of the related treatments discussed.

Ann Packman

Our group was interested from a clinical point of view how the therapist decides what to work on with parents. From my recall of the Demands and Capacities model there are four demands and four capacities, and the combination of them is different for each child. How does the clinician decide which of them is relevant to any child?

[1]Dave Rowley joined Mirjana Lasan to respond to the leaders of the discussion groups.

Mirjana Lasan

The parent essentially makes the decision. A video recording of children and parents interacting is made in the clinic and reviewed. Parents and clinicians watch the video, and the parent decides, guided by the clinician, what the targets for therapy should be. Parents determine what would be the best thing to enhance the child's fluency: whether, for example, they speak too fast or whether they ask too many questions. So together with parents they decide what would be the best thing to modify

Ann Packman

So then, if the initial choices did not produce any effects, the combination might be changed. Is that correct?

Mirjana Lasan

Yes, like any treatment, the entire process is constantly subject to potential revision.

Sheena Reilly

We had much discussion around the fact that there is limited evaluation for any of these styles of treatment, with small numbers of children. These treatments have been around for decades, so why do you think that more advanced and sophisticated clinical trials have never been done?

Dave Rowley

I think the answer is that these styles of treatment do not lend themselves to evaluation, because it is not perfectly clear what they are designed to attain. Hence, there has been no driving need to evaluate them. I think that is a shame because they may have real value. But if the question is posed 'What is the evidence that it works?', the only answer can be that there is limited evidence. The problem extends here to replication also, because the nature of the treatment is different for every child and that it is not fully clear what the treatment is designed to achieve. So it is difficult to imagine a future time when clinicians can be sure they are doing the same early intervention method that others have shown independently to be useful.

Joseph Attanasio

In terms of the Demands and Capacities model, perhaps we should look at capacity as performance. My reading of the approach suggests much emphasis on decreasing demand and but not much emphasis on increasing competence or performance. Perhaps it is just easier to decrease demand than to increase performance.

Mirjana Lasan

Definitely in my experience, in any treatment derived ultimately from multifactorial concepts, it is much easier to decrease demands. And that is why the clinical applications that I describe focus on just doing that.

Ann Packman

Another clinical question is that it is obvious, from the research that you presented, that some children will not respond to this style of treatment and will need a direct one. So when is the decision made to try a direct treatment?

Mirjana Lasan

Quite simply, when the indirect proves unsatisfactory.

Ann Packman

If they are still stuttering?

Mirjana Lasan

Yes.

Sheena Reilly

We were interested in a comment that you made about not making parents feel guilty and not adopting blame when using this sort of approach. We had much discussion about how do you manage to do that when what the clinician is really doing is removing parent behaviours that are implicated in the start and the continuation of stuttering.

Mirjana Lasan

Of course, feelings of guilt and blame might occur with all early stuttering interventions that involve the parents. I suppose that is the value of the parent education components of these treatments that tell parents about the multifactorial nature of what is happening and about how it is inevitable that this will trigger stuttering if a child is genetically prone to stuttering. With a proper clinical relationship with parents it should not be an issue.

Sheena Reilly

Surely then there must be a fine line there between being responsible and not being responsible for the child's stuttering, because the treatment focuses on behaviours they must stop doing in order to treat the stuttering. It must be a clinical challenge to get that just right.

Mirjana Lasan

You are absolutely correct that this is one of the challenges with presenting this treatment, particularly for junior clinicians who may be attempting it for the first time.

Joseph Attanasio

How do you handle the problem you mentioned that parents may not want to be involved in multifactorial treatment? They may, for example, just want the clinician to fix the problem during each clinic visit. It would be by definition impossible to do a multifactorial treatment without full parent involvement.

Mirjana Lasan

I do hope that I did not imply that such a problem was unique to any multifactorial style treatment. It is by definition a problem with any early intervention I know of that has been shown in any way to be empirically viable. Of course, on some occasions such an issue is a barrier to treatment, but fortunately most parents are not like that. Otherwise, I don't think early stuttering intervention would be possible.

References

Bernstein Ratner, N. (1992) Measurable outcomes of instructions to modify normal parent-child verbal interactions: implications for indirect stuttering therapy. *Journal of Speech and Hearing Research, 35*, 14-20.

Bernstein Ratner, N. (2004) Caregiver-child interactions and their impact on children's fluency: implications for treatment. *Language, Speech, and Hearing Services in Schools, 35*, 46-56.

Franken, M. C., Kielstra-Van der Schalka, C. J., & Boelens, H. (2005) Experimental treatment of early stuttering: a preliminary study. *Journal of Fluency Disorders, 30*, 189-199.

Guitar, B. (2006) *Stuttering: An Integrated Approach to its Nature and Treatment* (3rd ed.). Baltimore, MD: Lippincott Williams and Wilkins.

Kelman, E., Nicholas, A., & Millard, S. (2005) PCI 2005 (Parent-child interaction therapy). Workshop presented at 7th Oxford Dysfluency Conference, Oxford, England.

Meyers, S. C., & Freeman, F. (1985) Mother and child speech rates as a variable in stuttering and disfluency. *Journal of Speech and Hearing Research, 28*, 436-444.

Millard, S. K., Nicholas, A., & Cook, F. M. (2008) Is parent-child interaction therapy effective in reducing stuttering? *Journal of Speech, Language, and Hearing Research, 51*, 636-650.

Millard, S. K., Edwards, S., & Cook, F. M. (2009) Parent-child interaction therapy: adding to the evidence. *International Journal of Speech-Language Pathology, 11*, 61-76.

Newman, L., & Smit, A. (1989) Some effects of variations in response time latency on speech rate, interruptions, and fluency in children's speech. *Journal of Speech and Hearing Research, 2*, 635-644.

Packman, A., & Attanasio, J. S. (2004) *Theoretical Issues in Stuttering.* New York: Taylor & Francis.

Starkweather, C. W. (1987) *Fluency and Stuttering.* Englewood Cliffs, NJ: Prentice-Hall.

Rustin, L., Botterill, W., & Kelman, E. (1996) *Assessment and Therapy for Young Disfluent Children: Family Interaction.* San Diego, CA: Singular.

Yairi, E., & Ambrose, N. G. (1992) A longitudinal study of stuttering in children: a preliminary report. *Journal of Speech and Hearing Research, 35*, 755-760.

Yaruss, J. S., Coleman, C., & Hammer, D. (2006) Treating preschool children who stutter: description and preliminary evaluation of a family-focused treatment approach. *Language, Speech and Hearing Services in Schools, 37*, 118-136.

Yaruss, J. S., & Conture, E. G. (1995) Mother and child speaking rates and utterance lengths in adjacent fluent utterances - preliminary-observations. *Journal of Fluency Disorders, 20*(3), 257-278.

Zebrowski, P. M., Weiss, A. L., Savelkoul, E. M., & Hammer, C. S. (1996) The effect of maternal rate reduction on the stuttering, speech rates and linguistic productions of children who stutter: evidence from individual dyads. *Clinical Linguistics & Phonetics, 10*(3), 189-206.

Chapter 14

Cognitive Behaviour Therapy

Dave Rowley
De Montfort University, Leicester, UK

Overview

Cognitive Behaviour therapy (CBT) evolved from the coming together of behaviour therapy with cognitive therapy. Strictly speaking, CBT is not a distinct therapeutic technique, but an umbrella term encompassing several approaches, including but not limited to Rational Emotive Behaviour therapy, Rational Living therapy and Schema therapy. The core principle is that people's emotional reactions and behaviour are strongly influenced by cognitions: thoughts, beliefs and interpretations about themselves and the situations in which they find themselves. These cognitions give meaning to the events of their lives. CBT practitioners aim to treat problems such as dysfunctional emotions and unwanted behaviours by applying goal-oriented, systematic techniques to change the underlying cognitions. Lately CBT has been used in the treatment of people who stutter (PWS), mainly in helping them reduce associated anxiety and social avoidance, primarily with adults and adolescents.

What is the essence of CBT? The first stage is to develop a formulation of the problem. This is not a diagnosis, but an understanding of the problem, a picture of why the person is experiencing the problem, worked out jointly by the therapist and the client. The first stage in each session is to set an agenda and develop goals for the session and therapy as a whole. Typically patterns of unhelpful thinking will be examined and questioned. Clients would be encouraged to practice speaking in different situations and to examine and re-evaluate the negative thoughts they have about this. Clients are usually given tasks to do between sessions.

Theoretical basis

The behavioural component of CBT has its main roots in early work by Wolpe (1958), and the cognitive component has its roots with Beck (1975). Behaviour

The Science and Practice of Stuttering Treatment: A Symposium, First Edition. Edited by Suzana Jelčić Jakšić and Mark Onslow.

therapy was developed first, but just as behavioural psychology fell victim to the cognitive revolution in psychology, so did behaviour therapy. But behaviour therapy, rather than falling into disuse, merged, or perhaps more correctly became incorporated into, cognitive therapy.

One of the first pioneers of behaviour therapy was Mary Cover Jones. Her treatment of Peter's fear of a white rabbit using direct conditioning, in which a pleasant stimulus (food) was presented simultaneously with the rabbit, is one of the earliest uses of behavioural techniques in therapy (Jones, 1924). But it is Wolpe (1958) who has become best known for applying behavioural techniques to psychological problems, in particular his use of systematic desensitisation.

Aaron Beck, inspired by the work of Albert Ellis, was the leading developer of cognitive therapy (Beck, 1975), being initially particularly concerned with the treatment of depression. Later, he expanded his work to include anxiety disorders. Rachman (1997) details that during the 1980s and 1990s, the benefits of taking the aspects of each approach and combining them into one was recognised by, amongst others, David Clark in the United Kingdom and David Barlow in the United States, particularly in the treatment of panic disorders.

So why should CBT be used in the treatment of stuttering? Research by Stein et al. (1996) indicated that social anxiety disorder[1] as a problem secondary to stuttering may occur in at least 40% of PWS. More recently, Menzies et al. (2008) reported that 60% of their sample of 30 adults, who stuttered and sought treatment, met the DSM-IV (American Psychiatric Association, 1994) diagnostic criteria for social anxiety disorder. In addition, many of those who stutter will experience some degree of social anxiety even though it may fall short of the severity needed for a diagnosis of social anxiety. This anxiety and any accompanying social avoidance contribute to a significant amount of distress and dysfunction in the lives of PWS. It is here that the usefulness of CBT with PWS can be seen in its potential to reduce anxiety.

Demonstrated value

Cognitive behaviour therapists generally use an integrative, multi-system model to understand patients and plan treatment. Assessment centres primarily on cognitive and behavioural observations, but biological, interpersonal, social, spiritual and other factors may also be considered. The basic tenet is that there is a feedback loop between cognition and behaviour in which cognitive processes can influence behaviour, and behavioural change can influence cognitions.

In the treatment of anxiety disorders one of the basic methods is a gradual exposure to the actual, feared stimulus. The argument is that through

---

[1]Social anxiety disorder is another, more contemporary, term for social phobia.

exposure to the stimulus, this conditioning can be unlearned. Social anxiety disorder has often been treated with such exposure coupled with cognitive restructuring, as in Heimberg's group therapy protocol (Turk et al., 2001). A study by Clark et al. (2006), suggests that 62 patients meeting the DSM-IV criteria for social phobia improved more when treated with cognitive therapy than with exposure plus applied relaxation.

Hofmann and Smits (2008) conducted an extensive literature review of CBT studies comparing the efficacy of CBT versus a placebo for anxiety disorders. They reviewed from when records were available to March 2007. From an original 1165 studies identified, they found 27 that met their inclusion criteria, which were as follows:

(1) Clients had to be between ages 18 and 65 and have met DSM-III-R or DSM-IV diagnostic criteria for an anxiety disorder as determined by a psychometrically robust and structured diagnostic instrument.
(2) Clients had to be randomly assigned to either CBT or placebo. The placebo had to control for non-specific factors, such as regular contact with a therapist, reasonable rationale for the intervention and discussions of the psychological problem.
(3) The clinical severity of the anxiety disorder had to be assessed by means of psychometrically sound clinician-rated or self-report measures.
(4) Reports had to provide sufficient information to calculate effect sizes.

Support was found for the use of CBT in anxiety disorders. Specifically, the severity of anxiety symptoms was decreased for people who took CBT over placebo. For social anxiety disorder, the average effect size estimate (Hedges' g) was 0.62, the 95% CI was 0.39–0.86, with z value = 5.28, $p < 0.001$. According to Cohen (1969), an effect size of 0.6 equates to a medium effect, while McGraw and Wong (1992) suggested using a 'Common Language Effect Size' (CLES) statistic, which is the probability that a score sampled at random from one distribution will be greater than a score sampled from another. For the effect size here of 0.6, this translates into a CLES of 0.66. So if we randomly select one member at random from the CBT group and one from the placebo group, 66 times out of 100 the person from the CBT group will have a lower anxiety score. For this experiment this is a very acceptable result.

What evidence exists on the efficacy of CBT for social anxiety with stuttering? McColl et al. (2001) used a CBT package based on the cognitive restructuring programme for social phobia of Mattick et al. (1989), with 11 stuttering clients following referral for anxiety-related problems. All 11 had reportedly failed to successfully apply speech restructuring (see Preface for a definition of this term) skills in everyday situations, despite demonstrating fluency in the clinic. After 12 weekly 1-hour sessions of CBT, the participants showed significant reductions in the following measures: Fear of Negative Evaluation scale, State-Trait Anxiety Inventory Form Y-1 scores and Global Self-Rating of Stuttering Severity Scores. The former measures state anxiety levels, and the latter is a 9-point self-report measure of stuttering severity over the previous week. Unfortunately there was no comparison group nor did the study include follow-up assessments. Neither did it combine speech and psychological procedures.

Using the same CBT package, St Clare et al. (2009) reported outcomes following 5 days of intensive CBT. Twenty-six participants completed the Unhelpful Thoughts and Beliefs About Stuttering (UTBAS) checklist before and after the CBT. The UTBAS identifies negative intrusive thoughts experienced by adults who stutter. Mean UTBAS scores decreased significantly from pre-treatment to post-treatment, with every one of the 26 stuttering participants showing a reduction in scores following treatment. UTBAS scores reduced by an average of more than 40% and the effect size was extremely large at 2.5, suggesting clinical significance. Again, however, no comparison group was reported and there was no long-term follow-up. Another research group has reported a preliminary attempt to replicate these findings (Ezrati-Vinacour et al., 2007).

Ermes et al. (2008) examined the efficacy of group CBT on the severity of social anxiety as well as on co-morbid stuttering in 12 individuals suffering from both conditions. There was also a control group of people with social phobia who did not stutter. Following a routine 18 sessions of group CBT, there was a significant reduction in social phobia, (effect size = 1.10) but no change in either the subjective or objective measures of stuttering.

Menzies et al. (2008) conducted an experimental clinical trial of a CBT package for chronic stuttering. Thirty-two stuttering participants were randomly assigned to either a speech restructuring with CBT group (experimental) or a speech restructuring only group (control). The experimental group then immediately began a 10-week CBT programme. This was followed by 14 hours of speech restructuring treatment. CBT was presented before speech restructuring to enable evaluation of the effectiveness of CBT alone in reducing stuttering severity and anxiety. The control group received no treatment for approximately 10 weeks after randomisation, in line with the CBT treatment, and then began a speech restructuring programme identical to that of the experimental group. The findings at follow-up 12 months later showed that speech restructuring treatment on its own had no impact on the social phobia of the cohort. At the same follow-up time, participants who had received CBT showed no social phobia and had made greater improvements than control participants on a range of psychological measures of anxiety and avoidance. However, the CBT package made no difference to the stuttering frequency of those with or without social phobia.

Figure 14.1 shows the scores on the three primary outcome measures used in this trial before treatment and 12 months after completion of the speech treatment programme. Two of the three measures were statistically and clinically significant at that time: global assessment of functioning and percentage of fear hierarchy completed.

These studies then show the positive results of CBT on social anxiety. Unfortunately, several of them are lacking in a comparison group and are without long-term follow-up.

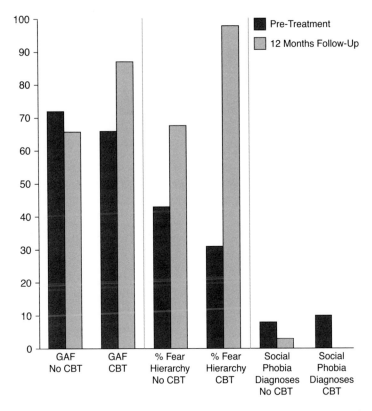

Figure 14.1   Mean results for participants in the Menzies et al. (2008) trial, showing participants who had CBT and those who did not 12 months after a speech restructuring treatment. Percentage fear hierarchy is the percentage of participants' fear hierarchy they reported completing. GAF, global assessment of functioning; CBT, cognitive behaviour therapy.

Advantages and disadvantages

Advantages

For PWS, it is clear that a compelling body of research exists in clinical psychology of potential benefits for PWS. Clinical trials to date are encouraging for the application of that body of information to PWS, although at present the evidence is limited. Subject numbers are small, long-term follow-up has not occurred and randomised evidence has been limited. However, as is the case for other applications, for PWS a short treatment of around 16 sessions seems sufficient to produce effects. There has been one attempt to design a CBT package specifically for the needs of PWS and are anxious.

Disadvantages

CBT depends critically on clients completing out-of-session tasks as directed by the clinician. If the client does not complete those tasks, then treatment success is not possible. Although this is a generally accepted limitation of CBT, with application to stuttering it is not an unusual limitation for speech and language therapy. There, the efficacy of any treatment depends on successful completion of prescribed activities by clients and their parents beyond the clinic.

CBT is an umbrella term including a number of therapies. Hence, there are a number of CBT packages each of which may have slightly different methods, such as duration of treatment, amount of out-of-session work and group or individual approach. This variety of different approaches within CBT makes it difficult to compare treatments, given that practitioners may be doing different things. However, a preliminary trial of a CBT package specifically for PWS may contribute to offsetting that problem for the future treatment of such clients.

Because CBT focuses on current negative appraisals and very specific cognitive-behavioural issues for the client, it does not always address the possible underlying causes of mental health conditions that might be driving such problems.

Conclusions and future directions

Preliminary research shows that CBT appears to be a promising method for reducing anxiety in clients who stutter. More and better research on its effectiveness in this group is needed. Unfortunately, it seems to have little direct affect on stuttering speech behaviour. Therefore, there is a need for research to establish which types of speech restructuring is the most effective match with CBT to reduce both social anxiety and stuttering speech behaviour.

CBT continues to develop in interesting ways. Currently, amongst the most prominent clinical models are those that focus particularly on the role of schemata in cognitive and behavioural difficulties. These have given rise to overtly schema-based approaches to cognitive therapy (Beck et al., 2004, Young, 1990). These include positive data logs (Padesky, 1994), which are systematically combined lists of positive experiences that are designed to build new, more constructive belief systems. Another development is continuum work or scaling (Pretzer, 1990), which is a strategy for helping people combat an unhelpful dichotomous thinking style.

Discussion

Joseph Attanasio

A basic question from our group. Despite many PWS meeting DSM-IV criteria for social phobia, is it really social phobia? Don't PWS have good reason to be anxious?[2] Are they really like others who are socially phobic but who don't stutter?

[2]The current version of the DSM-IV criteria (American Psychiatric Association, 1994) specifically excludes diagnosis of social phobia for those who stutter.

Dave Rowley

I think in terms of the way they present clinically, the answer is yes they are.

Sheena Reilly

What is your view of when CBT should be introduced? Do you think it should occur in concert with speech restructuring? Do you think it should be done before or do you think it should be done separately from speech restructuring? What implications might your answer have for the skill mix of the therapist or therapists?

Dave Rowley

A key issue here is that you work out a treatment agenda with the client. What happens during treatment is jointly constructed. It might emerge, for example, that the client wants to tackle speech restructuring straight away before CBT. I am not really aware of any evidence about which we should do first. But obviously, if the client needs and wants to work on anxiety first then of course that is what should be done.

Sheena Reilly

And the implications of that for the skill mix of the therapist?

Dave Rowley

I would argue that a speech and language therapist who deals with stuttering has the right background and therapeutic skills to learn how to use CBT. Courses to learn CBT are available from a number of sources. I am not a big fan of having those who stutter treated concurrently by speech-language therapists and psychologists. I think CBT should be part of the skill mix of speech and language therapists who deal with adults who stutter.

Ann Packman

Our group was interested in how long the effect of CBT lasts? So what's the evidence from the non-stuttering population and then what do you think about CBT with PWS?

Dave Rowley

The evidence in general is that its effects could be life long. But there is quite a lot of evidence of some relapsing cases that need further 'doses' of CBT. We don't know yet about whether that will be the case for stuttering, but my guess is it will be much the same. I do not see any theoretical reason why it should be any different.

Joseph Attanasio

The data show obvious improvement in terms of anxiety and avoidance, but not much in stuttering behaviour. Does the decrease in anxiety as a result of CBT actually translate into more talking despite stuttering?

Dave Rowley

There are two issues; whether they speak more in terms of word output or whether they go into previously avoided situations with comfort. The latter is one of the goals of CBT. I don't know of any evidence of whether that actually improves speech output in terms of an increase in words spoken.

Sheena Reilly

From what you said it seems a disadvantage of CBT for future clinical trials with stuttering, is that it cannot be a standardised package. What do you think are the implications of that for clinical trials?

Dave Rowley

I don't want to give the impression that there are no CBT package protocols to follow, because there are. But the issue is that many therapists will use one component only of CBT, not the entire package. There is a tendency to refer to having done CBT when in fact that is not really what occurred, parts of the package have been carried out but not all of it. I feel this makes it difficult to evaluate a body of clinical trials evidence that comes under the umbrella of CBT. So a positive development in our field is recent efforts to develop clearly documented CBT packages targeted specifically at those who stutter.

Ann Packman

We wanted to know whether the terms desensitisation and exposure during CBT are the same things and if not how do they differ?

Dave Rowley

I see them as being interchangeable terms referring to similar things. The origins of CBT are in the amalgamation of systematic desensitisation and cognitive therapy.

Ann Packman

So the challenges to cognitions are not desensitisation but the cognitive part of CBT. For example, 'Are people really laughing at you?' Is that correct?

Dave Rowley

Yes it is. That component of CBT is to have clients specify the faulty cognitions they are having and to get rid of them. Earlier attempts at systematic desensitisation did involve much thinking about the thoughts driving the problem itself, and also changing behaviour that resulted from it. So today, cognitive challenge and restructuring and systematic desensitisation are active components of CBT.

Joseph Attanasio

Does CBT also deal with unrealistic and unhelpful cognitions such as 'If I didn't stutter I could be the greatest trial lawyer in the world'?

Dave Rowley

Indeed it does. Clinical psychologists come across a range of people with different kinds of anxiety disorders who make the assumption that if it were not for their disorder then they would, as you say, 'be the greatest trial lawyer in the world', or whatever else they may think. Part of CBT is to help people come to a realistic position about their potential.

Sheena Reilly

We were intrigued by the findings that the anxiety reduction does not translate to reduced stuttering frequency. We thought it has long been assumed that anxiety and stuttering mediate each other. What do you think about that and why did anxiety reduction not lead to stuttering reduction?

Dave Rowley

I don't think I have a definitive answer to that, but I can tell you my thoughts about it. Anxiety is not a unitary phenomenon. Apart from the state-trait anxiety distinction that is well known, there are many components of anxiety that are not so commonly recognised. These include, for example, social avoidance and shyness. So in the first instance it may simply not be so straightforward to expect a relationship between general measures of 'anxiety' and stuttering rate. Perhaps part of the expectation that when anxiety reduces, stuttering will reduce is underpinned by an assumption that when anxiety increases stuttering will increase. That might be a reasonable, intuitive assumption, but as yet the research in support of it is scant (Ezrati-Vinacour and Levin, 2004; Gabel et al., 2002). But even if that is correct, it is not logical or scientific to expect the opposite effect. Considering the multi-faceted nature of stuttering as I just mentioned, when there is a positive correlation between stuttering and anxiety it is just not clear what variable or variables may have been responsible for that correlation. And even if it were clear, it would not be reasonable to expect them to have an effect in the opposite direction.

Sheena Reilly

Thank you, I think that is an important point.

Ann Packman

We were interested in the age range of people who may benefit from CBT. With those who stutter it seems clear that it can be done successfully with adults and young adults but do you think it could be used with children?

Dave Rowley

Indeed I know that one member of the group here has been using it with 9-year-old children. It seems to me that its not so much chronological age that is the crucial issue here, it is cognitive age and emotional age that is important. So I wouldn't want to say that it should only be used for children 13 and above, for example. I think if children are able to express their own thoughts and ideas then CBT is potentially useful. Children become able to talk about their internal feelings, anxieties and worries often at 8 or 9 years. So there is no reason in such cases why CBT would not be appropriate.

Joseph Attanasio

Do some stuttering clients object to the notion of CBT? We wondered if this could be a clinical problem because our speech pathology clients typically come to us wanting to focus on stuttering. They may anticipate speech therapy and then they are confronted with psychology.

Dave Rowley

Yes, I know exactly what you mean. Of course many who present for speech therapy have a goal to reduce stuttering and unexpectedly they are involved in psychology. However you package it, CBT is psychotherapy. It is enjoying better press now at least in the United Kingdom. But I am sure many people are not entirely sure what it is and how it is distinct from psychiatry. But of course if this were a potential clinical issue, then any competent speech-language therapist would be aware of it and address it with the client as needed.

References

American Psychiatric Association. (1994) *Diagnostic and Statistical Manual of Mental Disorders* (4th ed.). Washington, DC: American Psychiatric Association.

Beck, A. T. (1975) *Cognitive Therapy and the Emotional Disorders*. New York: International Universities Press Inc.

Beck, A. T., Freeman, A., Davis, D. D., & Associates (Eds.) (2004) *Cognitive Therapy of Personality Disorders* (2nd ed.). New York: Guildford Press.

Clark, D. M., Ehlers, A., Hackmann, A., McManus, F., Fennell, M., Grey, N., & Wild, J. (2006) Cognitive therapy versus exposure and applied relaxation in social phobia: a randomized controlled trial. *Journal of Consulting and Clinical Psychology, 74*, 568-578.

Cohen, J. (1969) *Statistical Power Analysis for the Behavioral Sciences*. New York: Academic Press.

Ermes, H., Marcom, S., & Hermesh, H. (2008) Effectiveness of cognitive behaviour group therapy in stutterers with generalized social phobia: therapeutic and diagnostic implications. *Journal of Affective Disorders, 107*(Supplement 1), S99.

Ezrati-Vinacour, R., & Levin, I. (2004) The relationship between anxiety and stuttering: a multidimensional approach. *Journal of Fluency Disorders, 29*, 135-148.

Ezrati-Vinacour, R., Gilboa-Schechtman, E., Anholt, G., Weizman, A., & Hermesh, H. (2007) Effectiveness of cognitive behaviour group therapy (CBGT) for social phobia (SP) in people who stutter (PWS) with social phobia (SP). Paper presented at the 5th World Congress of Behavioural and Cognitive Therapies.

Gabel, R. M., Colcord, R. D., & Petrosino, L. (2002) Self-reported anxiety of adults who do and do not stutter. *Perceptual and Motor Skills, 94*(3), 775-784.

Hofmann, S. G., & Smits, J. A. (2008) Cognitive-behavioral therapy for adult anxiety disorders: a meta-analysis of randomized placebo-controlled trials. *Journal of Clinical Psychiatry, 69*, 621-32.

Jones, M. C. (1924) A laboratory study of fear: the case of Peter. *Pedagogical Seminary, 31*, 308-315.

Mattick, R. P., Peters, L., & Clarke, J. C. (1989) Exposure and cognitive restructuring for social phobia: a controlled study. *Behaviour Therapy, 20*, 3-23.

McColl, T., Onslow, M., Packman, A., Menzies, R. G. (2001) A cognitive behavioural intervention for social anxiety in adults who stutter. Proceedings of the 2001 Speech Pathology Australia National Conference, Melbourne, Australia.

McGraw, K. O., & Wong, S. P. (1992) A common language effect size statistic. *Psychological Bulletin, 111*, 361-365.

Menzies, R. G., O'Brian, S., Onslow, M., Packman, A., St Clare, T., & Block, S. (2008) An experimental clinical trial of a cognitive-behavior therapy package for chronic stuttering. *Journal of Speech, Language, and Hearing Research, 51*, 1451-1464.

Padesky, C. A. (1994) Schema change processes in cognitive therapy. *Clinical Psychology and Psychotherapy, 1*, 267-278.

Pretzer, J. (1990) Borderline personality disorder. In: A. T. Beck, A. Freeman, D. Davis & Associates (Eds.), *Cognitive Therapy of Personality Disorders* (2nd ed., pp. 187-214). New York: Guildford Press.

Rachman, S. (1997) The evolution of cognitive behaviour therapy. In: D. Clark, C. G. Fairburn & M. G. Gelder (Eds.), *Science and Practice of Cognitive Behaviour Therapy*. Oxford: Oxford University Press.

St Clare, T., Menzies, R. G., Onslow, M., Packman, A., Thompson, R., & Block, S. (2009) Unhelpful thoughts and beliefs linked to social anxiety in stuttering: development of a measure. *International Journal of Language and Communication Disorders, 44*, 338-351.

Stein, M. B., Baird, A., & Walker, J. R. (1996) Social phobia in adults with stuttering. *American Journal of Psychiatry, 153*, 278-280.

Turk, C. L., Heimberg, R. G., & Hope, D. A. (2001) Social anxiety disorder. In: D. H. Barlow (Ed.), *Clinical Handbook of Psychological Disorders: A Step by Step Manual* (3rd ed., pp. 114-153). New York: Guilford Press.

Wolpe, J. (1958) *Psychotherapy by Reciprocal Inhibition*. Stanford, CA: Stanford University Press.

Young, J. E. (1990) *Cognitive Therapy for Personality Disorders: A Schema Focused Approach*. Saratosa, FL: Professional Resource Exchange.

Chapter 15
The Westmead Program

Natasha Trajkovski
The University of Sydney, Sydney, Australia

Overview

Stuttering is an imposing health care problem, with recent estimates of life-time risk of exposure around 10% (Bloodstein and Bernstein Ratner, 2008). The first prospective cohort study of stuttering onset confirmed by expert diagnosis, found a 36-month cumulative incidence of 8.6% (Reilly et al., 2009). Cumulative incidence at 46 months was 11.2% with only 6.3% of children recovering naturally during 12 months after onset (Reilly et al., 2011). Clinic-based estimates are typically lower. For example, Yairi et al. (1993) reported that 3 of 16 children (19%) had recovered from a clinic sample after 6 months. Regardless of what the correct figure may be, it is clear that many children who begin to stutter will still do so 12 months later, and most clinicians would commence treatment at 12 months post onset. In short, therefore, our profession simply does not have adequate resources to manage the public health problem of early stuttering. Accordingly, the development of a new treatment approach for preschool children, called the Westmead Program (WP), was commenced at the Australian Stuttering Research Centre. The purpose of this development was to explore a simpler and more cost effective treatment than those currently available. To date, Phase I and Phase II trials have shown considerable promise.

All that is required to conduct the WP is that children practise syllable-timed speech (STS) in conversation with their parents at regular intervals throughout the day. There are two stages to the programme. The aim of Stage 1 is to get children stutter free, and the aim of Stage 2 is to keep them stutter free whilst treatment is withdrawn.

During Stage 1, the child and parent attend the clinic to learn how to use STS in conversation. Then, they go home to practise the speech pattern together, four to six times per day for 5–10 minutes at a time. During the first clinic session, children are taught to use STS progressively, starting with imitation and working up through closed questions, open questions and finally into

The Science and Practice of Stuttering Treatment: A Symposium, First Edition. Edited by Suzana Jelčić Jakšić and Mark Onslow.
© 2012 John Wiley & Sons, Ltd. Published 2012 by John Wiley & Sons, Ltd.

conversation. It usually takes a preschooler 1 week of solid practice to maintain a 10-minute conversation with STS. During treatment, children may slip into and out of syllable use without consequence, other than praise for good 'robot talking', which is the term we normally used to describe STS to children. During Stage 1 of the WP, clinic visits are spaced weekly at first, until the child can use STS in conversation and then, once all the routine issues have been ironed out, visits are spaced fortnightly.

Progression criteria for Stage 2 of the WP are similar to the Lidcombe Program (LP) (see Chapter 4). Stage 2 begins when the child attains a within-clinic percent syllables stuttered (%SS) below 1.0 and a mean weekly beyond-clinic severity rating below 2.0 for 4 consecutive weeks. The structure of Stage 2 visits is also similar to the LP, as treatment is gradually withdrawn provided that the child's speech remains within the required stuttering criteria.

Theoretical basis

The WP is based on the well-known stuttering suppressor STS. STS involves speaking with minimal differentiation in linguistic stress across syllables and is achieved by saying each syllable in time to a rhythm. This procedure has been known for centuries as being among the most powerful agents for the control of stuttering (Bloodstein, 1987; Ingham, 1984; Van Riper, 1973; Wingate, 1976). However, as is the case with all such agents, it is not fully clear at present how STS controls stuttering.

Not surprisingly for such a marked speech pattern, many acoustic, linguistic and aerodynamic changes have been identified when speakers use STS. As such, there have been many potential theoretical explanations for the STS effect. One simple explanation is that STS aids the timing of speech production (Van Riper, 1973). Another explanation is that STS provides a distraction from stuttering (Azrin et al., 1968; Brady, 1969). Andrews et al. (1983) related the STS effect to sensory and motor speech adjustments, and Harrington (1987, 1988) put forward that somehow STS enables real time correction of auditory speech regulation. More recently, it has been proposed that STS reduces or eliminates linguistic stress, which in turn eliminates a trigger for stuttering (Packman et al., 2000).

Regardless of why it might work, it is well known that the remedial effects of STS on stuttering are only temporary in adults, lasting only for as long as the speech pattern can be maintained. This is presumably because, by adulthood, the neural pathways for speech have already become established (Craig and Hancock, 1995; Wohlert and Smith, 2002). With children however, neural pathways for speech are still being laid down and long-term changes in the speech mechanism may still be possible (Packman et al., 2000). It is this line of reasoning that has driven the development of the WP; that a brief period of STS use during early childhood may provide lasting, effortless and undetectable control of stuttering.

Despite its clear theoretical promise, research into the use of STS to treat early stuttering has been limited, probably because of the unsatisfactory results obtained with adults. In fact, there have been only three reports of STS used to treat children. Of these, only one study reported on preschool children (Coppola and Yairi, 1982), whilst the other two studies reported on school-age children (Alford and Ingham, 1969; Andrews and Harris, 1964). All three studies convey a uniform result of positive but limited responsiveness to STS being taught using a metronome and programmed instruction. Arguably, at least with preschool children, better results may be obtained if programmed instruction were removed. In fact, one report suggests that programmed instruction may not even be necessary to obtain a treatment effect. Greenburg (1970) conducted an experiment suggesting that STS may control the stuttering of children simply with exposure.

Demonstrated value

Using the Onslow et al. (2008) definition of a clinical trial,[1] there have been three preliminary clinical trials of the WP. Initially, outcomes were reported for the treatment in a single case study (Trajkovski et al., 2006). In that study, a 3-year 2-month-old boy was treated. Independent, blinded measures showed that 7 clinic visits over 21 weeks were required for the child to reach the criteria for progression into Stage 2.

Subsequently, the responses of three children to the treatment were reported using a multiple baseline design across three participants (Trajkovski et al., 2009). Independent, blinded measures showed that the children required a mean of 8.6 clinic visits over 18 weeks to attain a beyond-clinic %SS below 1.0. The first participant was a 3-year 5-month-old girl, the second a 3-year 11-month-old boy and the third a 3-year 8-month-old boy. All three children reached a beyond-clinic %SS below their pre-treatment baseline levels. It was clear that reductions of beyond-clinic %SS for all children were evident only after the introduction of treatment. However, only one child completed the treatment; the other two dropped out because they reached a plateau in severity, which prevented them from progressing into Stage 2. In other words, the STS practice alone was not enough for these two children to control their stuttering to satisfactory levels, only to bring it close to those levels.

The most compelling clinical trials data for the WP at present, albeit preliminary, is a non-randomised Phase II trial. Seventeen preschool children were recruited at a mean age of 3 years 8 months. %SS was the primary outcome and was measured from beyond-clinic recordings by a blinded independent observer. Eight children completed the trial with a mean pre-treatment %SS of 6.0, and at 12 months post Stage 2 entry, their beyond-clinic %SS scores were 0.2. These results were obtained in a mean of 8.0 clinician hours, which is around half the mean hours required to complete Stage 1 of the LP. The dropout rate was 52.9%, which is substantive, but is comparable to the mean of 42.6% for published trials with stuttering preschoolers. Figure 15.1 shows the results for the individual children.

[1]A prospective attempt to determine the efficacy of an entire treatment based on at least 3 months follow-up observations of speech beyond the clinic.

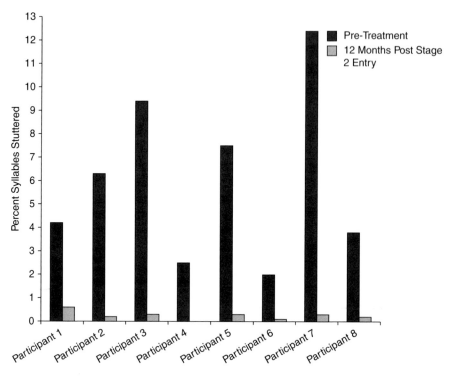

Figure 15.1 Percent syllables stuttered pre-treatment and at 12 months entry to Stage 2 for the eight children who completed the trial.

It is important with a treatment that uses a novel speech pattern to be sure that speech is not in any way unusual sounding. So we assembled random post-treatment recordings, 15 seconds in duration, and had non-clinicians listen to them. We instructed them to write down words or phrases that described the samples. None of the words they wrote suggested there was anything unusual sounding about the children's speech.

Advantages and disadvantages

Advantages

From the Phase II trial results, the WP appears to require minimal clinic contact in order to achieve what we generally accept as clinically satisfactory stuttering control. Not only were clinic visits quite short in duration, with only half an hour needed to complete each scheduled appointment, but clinic visits were also spaced fortnightly for most of Stage 1.

The treatment is also suitable for very young children. With the LP at least, intervention at this age is not advisable because responsiveness appears to depend to some extent on the cognitive development of the child. This is inferred by recovery plot analyses showing treatment to take longer when onset-to-treatment time is shorter (Kingston et al., 2003). However, given evidence that children as young as 3 years may experience negative conse-quences as a result of their stuttering (Ezrati-Vinacour et al., 2001; Langevin et al., 2009), the need for suitable interventions for that age is pressing.

It is also the case that the WP protocol is straightforward. Participants are only required to practise STS for around 1 cumulative hour per day and have their daily severity scores recorded by their parents. It is also the case that verbal contingencies, particularly those for stuttered speech, raise safety issues. Without the need for verbal contingencies, such fundamental questions of safety may be avoided altogether. It may be the case, however, that the treatment has optimal effects when verbal contingencies are incorporated into it (see Section Conclusions and future directions).

Finally, and perhaps most significantly, given the inherent simplicity of the treatment, it may be possible for the WP to be safely modified and deliv-ered with more cost efficient models, hence increasing health care efficiency and decreasing treatment costs. Those treatment models could include group treatment and stand-alone Internet treatment.

Disadvantages

The Phase II trial has demonstrated that the WP, in its current form, needs some revision. Even though the speech outcomes are positive, a significant rate of withdrawal was associated with the preliminary version of the pro-gramme. Although dropouts are common for this type of research, they are nonetheless concerning. Most families ceased treatment because of some ex-tenuating family circumstance. In reality though, many of these families would have continued with treatment if the speech gains made were worth the effort required to continue treatment despite their difficult circumstances. This was not the case, as all nine children who withdrew from treatment had reached a plateau in severity, just above programme criteria, which prevented them from progressing to Stage 2.

Conclusions and future directions

There is a need for an efficacious and simple treatment that can be used with very young stuttering children. Clinical results so far are encouraging and we have begun a randomised controlled trial comparing the WP to the LP. When that trial is complete we will know whether we have access to such an efficacious and simple treatment, and whether we attain further efficiency improvements with group and Internet presentations of it.

Given that most children dropped out of our Phase II trial at the point when low-level stuttering severity plateaued slightly above target criteria, we spec-ulated that further speech gains may be achieved through the application of verbal contingencies for stuttered and stutter-free speech. To conduct this hy-brid version of the programme, parents were required to carry out a standard 'robot talking' practise session for 5-10 minutes and then immediately switch a to 'smooth talking' practice session for another 5-10 minutes. During 'smooth talking' practice, the child reverts to customary speech and is given feedback about speech performance, in the same way as with the LP. The advantage of conducting a 'robot talking' session immediately beforehand is that fluency can be carried over and parents do not have to manipulate language output to maintain the correct praise to correction ratio. Once verbal contingencies are mastered during structured practise, parents are then taught to add them to unstructured conversation.

By integrating verbal contingencies into the WP, we hope that children may become better equipped to reduce their stuttering past the point at which STS use is efficient. In fact, it is reasonable to foresee that the addition of verbal contingencies to the WP may serve as a valuable second step in a schedule of stepped care[2] for children who may otherwise withdraw from treatment for lack of progress or for parents who burn out. We have now completed testing this new WP protocol and have begun a three-arm randomised trial to compare the WP, the LP and the hybrid treatment.

Discussion

Sheena Reilly

We were interested in the dropout rate and the reasons the parents gave for withdrawing from the study and we wondered if that said something about the acceptability of the programme for the parents. Perhaps their kids were just better enough and they did not need to do any more treatment.

Natasha Trajkovski

Most kids did drop out at a very low severity, even though it was in fact above programme criteria. So, I can understand that parents would be satisfied with that outcome and would not want to keep on going, because it is quite an intensive treatment to conduct at home. For them, it was a case of near enough was good enough.

Joseph Attanasio

We also had a question about dropouts. It was quite a large percentage, and possibly the remaining children did in fact remain because they were naturally recovering. In other words, the dropouts might have been the children who did not respond at all well and were not naturally recovering, and the ones you retained were retained for the very reason they were naturally recovering.

Natasha Trajkovski

Of course, natural recovery is always an issue with clinical trials of early stuttering treatments. That is why we did a multiple baseline study: to be

[2]The Stepped Care model of health care delivery contains two fundamentals (Bower and Gilbody, 2005). It provides the simplest and most cost efficient method of health care that is efficacious. It is self-correcting so that patients progressively escalate to more resource intensive, and less cost efficient, health care models if they are shown to need it. It is suitable for disorders where simple, cost efficient interventions can be used for a significant proportion of those affected, such as brief counselling for weight control or management of substance abuse.

sure, at least with those three kids, that it was the treatment that caused the improvements.

Sheena Reilly

We have a question about how the parent and/or the family are involved. The parent comes to each clinic visit and then models STS. Is that all they do? Do they give feedback to the children about their STS?

Natasha Trajkovski

The parents come into the clinic and I sit down with them and ask them to show me what they are doing at home. Then they model 'robot talking' to the child and just by hearing the model, the child will usually slip into robot talking. If the child doesn't slip into robot talking, the parent can simply ask the child to use the pattern. But we don't like to encourage that because it can tend to be punitive if overused. A better idea is for the parent to start off with closed questioning, which elicits shorter sentences, and then the child is more likely to maintain robot talking.

Sheena Reilly

Does the parent give praise for using robot talking?

Natasha Trajkovski

Yes, the parent says something like 'good robot talking' when they hear robot talking. If they don't hear robot talking, they don't say anything. If the child stutters, they don't say anything.

Ann Packman

Could you talk a little bit about LP versus WP, particularly in relation to the age of the child? We understand that they are doing quite different clinical things, but you also talked about future combination of LP features into the WP. The group wondered about the ages for which the two treatments might be suitable, and the age that would most benefit from the hybrid treatment.

Natasha Trajkovski

The youngest child that I have treated with the WP was 36 months. With the LP, treatment at that young age is generally thought not advisable because the treatment depends on some level of cognitive development. The WP is so simple that cognitive maturity isn't an issue. Regarding the hybrid treatment, we have no idea at all as yet when or under what circumstances that treatment might be more suitable.

Joseph Attanasio

Our thinking was that perhaps what you're doing is helping the child through some difficulty with dealing with the demands of processing variable linguistic stress that might trigger stuttering as described by the Vmodel (Packman et al., 1996).

Natasha Trajkovski

Yes, I agree. The Vmodel and its potential role with early stuttering treatment was discussed by Packman et al. (2000).

Ann Packman

Some of our group were surprised at how natural the children sounded.[3] How long does it take in your clinical experience to go from the 'choppy robot' talking to when they first start to sound quite natural?

Natasha Trajkovski

Children only use robot talking during the treatment time itself. Once treatment concludes, children will revert back to customary, natural-sounding speech immediately and spontaneously.

Ann Packman

Returning to the dropout rate, it appears related to meeting the criteria for Stage 1 so that children can progress to Stage 2. Would that be right?

Natasha Trajkovski

Yes, almost but not quite reaching the criteria.

Ann Packman

So our question was, do you think the criteria are too strict? Are you asking too much of the children?

Natasha Trajkovski

I don't think so. We are asking the same as the LP, which for our purposes are a gold standard for control of early stuttering. The only way we can compare it to the LP, either indirectly with clinical benchmarks or directly in clinical trials, is to use the same criteria.

Ann Packman

But do you think given the dropout rate that that is asking too much? Is it a treatment component that could be manipulated? Could you reduce or make the treatment less intensive for children that are not progressing straight to criteria in the hope of reducing the dropout rate?

Natasha Trajkovski

That strikes me as counter-intuitive in terms of treatment efficacy. If anything, I would do more intensive treatment to get them to Stage 2. I don't think reducing treatment intensity will solve the dropout problem. Perhaps a stepped care approach will solve the dropout problem, when children fail to quickly attain Stage 2 criteria with the WP the hybrid programme is next.

Joseph Attanasio

On that topic, praising robot talking is a verbal contingency. Would the other contingency then be a correction of not using the robot speech?

Natasha Trajkovski

No, the same verbal contingencies that are used in the LP would be used in the hybrid version.

---

[3]Dr Trajkovski showed the group some pre-treatment and post-treatment videos of children during the Westmead clinical trials.

Joseph Attanasio

Would that not confound the effects of STS? Those contingencies have been shown to be quite potent in laboratory studies.

Natasha Trajkovski

And that's why we are including them.

Joseph Attanasio

That would complicate the treatment.

Natasha Trajkovski

Yes, and that is why we would introduce them as the second step in a stepped care sequence.

Sheena Reilly

When would you introduce the contingencies for stuttered and stutter-free speech? What will be your criteria for doing that?

Natasha Trajkovski

We have set a criterion that if severity ratings do not fall for 8 consecutive weeks, contingencies are introduced. When introducing contingencies, we keep them separate from the 'robot talking' practice. So, we have parents do 'robot talking' practice first as usual for 5-10 minutes, and then we get them to immediately switch to the LP verbal contingencies. That way, we plan to maximise carry over from WP treatment benefits to LP treatment benefits.

Ann Packman

The practise requirements of four to six times a day for 5-10 minutes. We were wondering if you could tell us why you chose those particular times.

Natasha Trajkovski

For two reasons. First, preschoolers just can't concentrate for much longer than 5-10 minutes at a time. Second, from a theoretical perspective, it makes sense that more bursts of STS practice would be better than fewer.

Joseph Attanasio

The image of a robot is strong and powerful. Is it necessary or helpful?

Natasha Trajkovski

I have never thought about that. It is of course arbitrary how you refer to the speech pattern. I guess we just fell into the habit of having parents use the 'robot talking' term. One mother I know of calls it 'syllable talking' and that did not seem to make a difference.

Sheena Reilly

What do parents think of this robot talking?

Mother[4]

I found the treatment sort of really easy to get a handle on...and also really easy for HM to do...this robot talking...was really sort of simple and

---

[4]Dr Trajkovski then played a video recorded interview with a parent whose child had been successfully treated with the WP. An excerpt of what she said is reproduced here.

straightforward...we would just have to practise speaking in a robot-like voice together for several minutes and that's all that was involved...He loved it. He especially liked coming here and he actually quite enjoyed the idea of speaking like a robot.

Natasha Trajkovski
To finish up, I would say that parents do generally like the treatment. They find it easy to learn, but the one thing that parents can have difficulty with is scheduling so many practice sessions. We have next to solve the problem of when that causes non-compliance.

References

Alford, J., & Ingham, R. (1969) The application of a token reinforcement system to the treatment of stuttering in children. *Journal of the Australian College of Speech Therapists, 19,* 53-57.

Andrews, G., & Harris, M. (1964) *The Syndrome of Stuttering.* London, UK: Heinemann.

Andrews, G., Craig, A., Feyer, A. M., Hoddinot, S., Howie, P., & Neilson, M. (1983) Stuttering: a review of research findings and theories circa 1982. *Journal of Speech and Hearing Disorders, 48,* 226-246.

Azrin, N., Jones, R. J., & Flye, B. (1968) A synchronization effect and its application to stuttering by a portable apparatus. *Journal of Applied Behavioral Analysis, 1,* 283-295.

Bloodstein, O. (1987) *A Handbook on Stuttering* (4th ed.). Chicago, IL: National Easter Seal Society.

Bloodstein, O., & Bernstein Ratner, N. (2008) *A Handbook on Stuttering.* Clifton Park, NY: Delmar.

Bower, P., & Gilbody, S. (2005) Stepped care in psychological therapies: access, effectiveness and efficiency. *The British Journal of Psychiatry, 186,* 11-17.

Brady, J. P. (1969) Studies on the metronome effect on stuttering. *Behavior Research and Therapy, 7,* 197-205.

Coppola, V., & Yairi, E. (1982) Rhythmic speech training with preschool stuttering children: an experimental study. *Journal of Fluency Disorders, 7,* 447-457.

Craig, A. R., & Hancock, K. (1995) Self-reported factors related to relapse following treatment for stuttering. *Australian Journal of Human Communication Disorders, 23,* 48-60.

Ezrati-Vinacour, R., Platzky, R., & Yairi, E. (2001) The young child's awareness of stuttering-like disfluency. *Journal of Speech, Language, and Hearing Research, 44,* 368-380.

Greenburg, J. B. (1970) The effect of a metronome on the speech of young stutterers. *Behaviour Therapy, 1,* 240-244.

Harrington, J. (1987) A model of stuttering and the production of speech under delayed auditory feedback. In: H. Peters & W. Hulstijn (Eds.), *Speech Motor Dynamics in Stuttering* (pp. 353-359). New York, NY: Springer-Verlag.

Harrington, J. (1988) Stuttering, delayed auditory feedback, and linguistic rhythm. *Journal of Speech and Hearing Research, 31,* 36-47.

Ingham, R. J. (1984) *Stuttering and Behavior Therapy: Current Status and Experimental Foundations.* San Diego, CA: College-Hill Press.

Kingston, M., Huber, A., Onslow, M., Jones, M., & Packman, A. (2003) Predicting treatment time with the LP: replication and meta-analysis. *International Journal of Language and Communication Disorders, 38*, 165–177.

Langevin, M., Packman, A., & Onslow, M. (2009) Peer responses to stuttering in the preschool setting. *American Journal of Speech-Language Pathology, 18*, 264–278.

Onslow, M., Jones, M., O'Brian, S., Menzies, R., & Packman, A. (2008) Defining, identifying, and evaluating clinical trials of stuttering treatments: a tutorial for clinicians. *American Journal of Speech-Language Pathology, 17*, 401–415.

Packman, A., Onslow, M., & Menzies, R. (2000) Novel speech patterns and the control of stuttering. *Disability and Rehabilitation, 22*, 65–79.

Packman, A., Onslow, M., Richard, F., & VanDoorn, J. (1996) Syllabic stress and variability: a model of stuttering. *Clinical Linguistics and Phonetics, 10*, 235–263.

Reilly, S., Onslow, M., Packman, A., Cini, E., Conway, L., Ukoumunne, O., & Block, S. (2011) Predicting stuttering onset and recovery by 4 years of age in a community-ascertained cohort. Manuscript in preparation.

Reilly, S., Onslow, M., Packman, A., Wake, M., Bavin, E., Prior, M., Eadie, P., Cini, E., Bolzonello, C., & Ukoumunne, O. (2009) Predicting stuttering onset by age 3 years: a prospective, community cohort study. *Pediatrics, 123*, 270–277.

Trajkovski, N., Andrews, C., O'Brian, S., Onslow, M., & Packman, A. (2006) Treating stuttering in a preschool child with syllable timed speech: a case report. *Behaviour Change, 23*, 270–277.

Trajkovski, N., Andrews, C., Onslow, M., Packman, A., O'Brian, S., & Menzies, R. (2009) Using syllable-timed speech to treat preschool children who stutter: a multiple baseline experiment. *Journal of Fluency Disorders, 34*, 1–10.

Van Riper, C. (1973) *The Treatment of Stuttering.* Englewood Cliffs, NJ: Prentice Hall.

Wingate (1976) *Stuttering Theory and Treatment.* New York, NY: Irvington Publishers.

Wohlert, A. B., & Smith, A. (2002) Developmental change in variability of lip muscle activity during speech. *Journal of Speech, Language, and Hearing Research, 45*, 1077–1087.

Yairi, E., Ambrose, N. G., & Niermann, R. (1993) The early months of stuttering - A developmental study. *Journal of Speech and Hearing Research, 36*, 521–528.

Chapter 16

Conscious Synthesis of Development: A Holistic Approach to Stuttering

Jelena Tadić and Darinka Šoster

Institute for Psychological Disorders and Speech Pathology, Belgrade, Serbia

Overview

Conscious synthesis of development (CSD) treatment is divided into three phases with well-defined and established activities that emphasise practising various skills, starting from least to the most demanding ones (Brajović and Brajović, 1976, 1981). The CSD treatment focuses with the client on problems of remediable psychological and belief disorders and physiological problems. Examples include biological rhythms, voice problems, avoidance behaviour, negative feelings and attitudes towards stuttering and other existing problems. To cover all this, the current approach incorporates different techniques aiming at sensory integration, attention and time tracking skills, fluency shaping and elements of cognitive-behavioural therapy.

Brajović had a very rigorous approach to therapy; clients were given very clear rules, which applied to many situations. General rules included getting enough sleep and eating regularly. It was also emphasised that clients must not deviate from the therapeutic principles they were given and that daily practice was a critical part of the therapy. There was also a focus on positive thinking; clients were encouraged to visualise speaking successfully in a variety of different situations. The endpoint of therapy was also clearly defined, as were the criteria for moving from one stage to another and once clients had successfully learned a technique, they were encouraged to teach it to others. In fact, being able to teach it to others was one of the criteria for measuring success. The role of parents was important too; particularly the mother, and they were expected to act as a therapist for the client. For older clients a significant other, usually the spouse, took the role of a therapist.

The Science and Practice of Stuttering Treatment: A Symposium, First Edition. Edited by Suzana Jelčić Jakšić and Mark Onslow.
© 2012 John Wiley & Sons, Ltd. Published 2012 by John Wiley & Sons, Ltd.

Since Brajović's times, the CSD approach has been modified and supplemented based on the development of cognitive behaviour therapy, as well as on clinical experience and client feedback. With certain modifications, this method is suitable for a wide range of clients, from preschool children to adults who stutter. Today, all Brajović's postulates for CSD therapy mentioned previously still apply, but due to changed life demands during recent decades, we are not so rigorous with some of the demands anymore. The CSD method today still emphasises on increased sensory awareness to facilitate the client's ability to correct behaviours. Hence, the client addresses all the steps involved in speaking: from formulating an idea to overt speech. This therapy approach to stuttering was of great influence across the former Yugoslavia and beyond (Fibiger et al., 2008; Jelčić, 1992; Jelčić Jakšić, 2002; Jelčić Jakšić et al., 2002; Podbrežnik and Čepelnik, 2002, 2010).

Assessment and therapy

The management process starts with an evaluation made by a speech-language pathologist and psychologist, and if needed by other members of the team including a neurologist and psychiatrist. This multidisciplinary approach is seen as a crucial element in the assessment and treatment of the client. Then, the goals of the final outcome are determined. They are set together by the therapist and client or his/her parents in the case of stuttering children, as family members are to take an active part in the treatment. They are all introduced to some general rules and suggestions that can help the client in achieving set goals and which relate to sleeping, nutrition and daily routine. To meet these goals, the therapist, within reason, adapts activities to the individual needs of the client. Specifically, age, other potentially existing speech-language problems, personal interests of the client and any other relevant issues are considered.

The client is strongly encouraged to practise daily and family members and friends are seen as an important part of treatment, and the importance of taking an active role in the treatment is clearly explained to them. If needed, the therapist will contact or personally visit the preschool or other social setting where the client spends a lot of time.

The treatment has three Phases and in each new phase what has already been learned is still practised.

Phase I

Phase I occurs at the outpatient unit one to three times per week. It involves practicing and mastering basic speech techniques such as breathing, voicing with easy onset and controlling voice pitch and facial muscles. Phase I also involves practising attention, concentration and time tracking skills. Also during this stage, clients learn to integrate verbal and non-verbal communication skills such as eye contact and positive facial expression. Finally, clients learn to overcome blocks.

Phase II

Phase II also occurs at the outpatient unit one to three times per week, but during this phase clients can also be admitted for residential therapy. During Phase II, clients practise and master advanced speech techniques and learn to apply them in moderately complex speech contexts: pronouncing connected words, phrasing and pausing in reading and story retelling. Clients create a hierarchy of difficult real life speech situations as well as a hierarchy of listener reactions that trigger negative emotional reactions and general distress during conversations. Clients learn and practice relaxation techniques with a focus on imagining the difficult speech situations from the hierarchy during relaxation. These imagined speech situations are dealt with in the safe therapy environment followed by an analysis of the behaviour. In addition, clients may participate in a residential group treatment.

Phase III

The essential elements of Phase III are working on conversation, interpersonal interaction and real life situations. It consists of several different components, which usually include a 2-week residential period and group and individual therapy at the outpatients unit. Generally, residential treatment does not occur at the start of this phase. The usual initial format is group therapy and individual sessions according to need. Clients move into real life situations for the purpose of desensitisation. This is intended to sharpen the client's capacity to consciously anticipate impending stuttering moments during communication. Phase III enables clients to take control over their speech in everyday life by learning to selectively use learned speech techniques and elements of cognitive behaviour therapy as needed. Gradually, the role of the therapist diminishes and clients become their own therapists.

Residential therapy

During the 14 days of the residential component, 8–12 clients are treated. Preschool children as young as 6.5 years can be included in this residential setting. Family members are encouraged to reside as well as the clients. Days 2–12 of the residential component involve group treatment, including elements of Phase II and III. If needed, additional individual sessions are scheduled, with the goal of overcoming other speech, language or other co-morbid problems.

The first and last day of group residential therapy includes evaluation of speech disfluencies, the subjective distress experienced in typical speech situations, the subjective distress caused by listener reactions to stuttering and personal attitudes towards stuttering.

Follow-up and maintenance

After Phase III clients return to the outpatient unit for follow-up and maintenance. They are again strongly encouraged to continue to practice daily. Follow-up and maintenance include individual and group sessions with elements of both Phase II and Phase III, with an increasing time period be-tween sessions. There are four types of clients who may be offered additional residential treatments. First, those who come to the maintenance and par-ticipate as co-therapists and role models for newcomers. Second, those who need prolonged treatment due to the severity of their problems. Third, those who live too far away to come to the outpatient unit for follow-up and main-tenance sessions. Finally, further residential treatment might be offered for clients who relapse after a long period post-treatment.

Theoretical basis

Stuttering is generally viewed today as a complex multifactorial disorder that affects the person as a whole, in which a combination of genetic, physiologi-cal, psychological and environmental factors can cause, trigger and modulate the occurrence, frequency, severity and maintenance of stuttering (Ambrose, 2008; Archibald and De Nil, 1999; De Nil et al., 2001; Dobrota-Davidović et al., 2007; Eggers et al., 2010; Guitar, 2006; Namasivayam and van Lieshout, 2008; Simić-Ružić and Jovanović, 2008; Tadić et al., 2009; Watkins et al., 2008). This realisation forces well-informed clinicians to come up with treat-ments addressing the different aspects of stuttering.

Starting from this multidimensional view of humans and bearing in mind the diverse symptomatology in people who stutter, Brajović and Brajović (1976, 1981) developed the CSD method, or Svesna Sinteza Razvoja in Serbian, which was a synthesis of the approaches to stuttering current at that time (Beck, 1975; Van Riper, 1973; Wolpe, 1958). The name comes from the approach taken to address holistically the person who stutters (Brajović et al., 2010).

Within the original CSD approach it was assumed that disorders such as stut-tering can be overcome, but also that one cannot change them if clients are not fully aware of them. This is why it was postulated that, first, the disordered functions must be consciously identified and people who stutter must become aware of their physiological and psychological functioning and relevant en-vironmental factors through sensations, feelings and behaviours. Second, by copying the natural development of these functions, they are consciously de-veloped or returned to the level they were at before stuttering occurred, in other words, to an adequate way of functioning. The client uses conscious awareness to integrate these newly developed or redeveloped functions in a harmonious interplay.

Demonstrated value

Expected therapy outcomes differ for different clients. In most cases, the ex-pected outcome is to achieve a significant decrease in all aspects of stuttering. The aim of therapy is for the client to take control over their speech and to be satisfied with their functioning in most speech situations.

In the 1970s there was research done with the approval of the US gov-ernment, which showed that the method is successful in dealing with speech

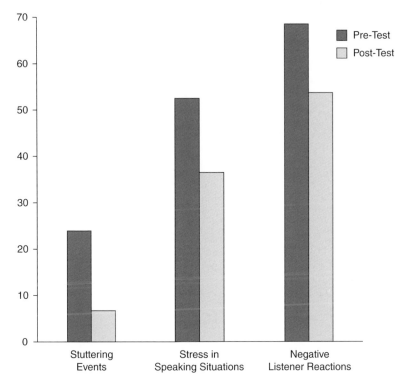

Figure 16.1 Mean initial and final mean scores for 140 conscious synthesis of development (CSD) clients in residential treatment. Number of stuttering events during 300 spoken words in reading, retelling, enumerating and conversation. Mean subjective units of distress scores for 18 common speaking situations. Mean subjective units of distress scores for Stress caused by listener reaction during 13 common speaking situations.

and concomitant problems in clients who strictly followed the methodology (Brajović and Brajović, 1981; Brajović et al., 2010). The research stressed the importance of parents and other significant people being included in the therapy. Recently, we have been conducting new research and our data so far also show that most of our clients benefited greatly from the programme (Šoster, 2003; Šoster et al., 2007; Tadić et al., 2010). The data here include these sources and in addition, recent data from one group of 140 clients, which has not been previously published.[1] These are file audit data taken from routine CSD treatments. Some clients do not return for treatment after initial diagnostics, and some clients do not complete their treatment. We present only data for those clients who completed treatment.

The initial data that are presented in Figure 16.1 were collected not at pre-treatment but during the first day of residential therapy, at which time clients' stuttering had decreased because they had attained some control over their

---

[1]Although it is not standard practice to publish data at two sources, we felt that it should occur here for the benefit of English speaking readers who otherwise would not have access to data in Serbian language publications.

speech. The final data were collected on the final day of residential treatment. Most of the data are from clients during Phase II.

In Figure 16.1, the number of stuttering events were based on 300 words spoken in the clinic while reading, retelling, enumerating and conversation. The stuttering events were counted in real time by a clinician. The subjective distress in situations is based on a list of 18 common speaking situations (Šoster, 2003). Clients use a 100-point Subjective Units of Distress scale based on Wolpe (1969) and refined by Radonjić (1982): '0' means 'total peace' and '100' means 'state of panic', meaning that the client is incapable of being in that situation. For each of the 18 situations, clients assign a Subjective Units of Distress score, and a mean score is established for each client. The mean of scores for clients is presented in Figure 16.1. The stress caused by listener reaction is a similar scale of 13 common listener reactions (Tadić et al., 2010), which is again scored with the Subjective Units of Distress measure. For the latter two scales, all clients are invited to make them shorter or much longer, depending on their own experiences.

All measures showed reductions of scores from initial to final assessment. Number of stuttering events dropped by 73%, which was the greatest outcome improvement. Distress in speech situations dropped by 44%. Spontaneous speech, taking an oral exam, reading and story retelling to strangers were the most difficult situations, both initially and at the end of treatment. Speaking to the clinician and enumerating were the easiest tasks, again both at the beginning and end of treatment. Stress caused by listener reaction dropped by 22%. The highest level of distress was caused by listener insults, laughter, ridicule and imitation, while clients experienced the least stress when their listeners made positive inquiries.

Advantages and disadvantages

Advantages

An advantage of the CSD treatment is that the method can cover a broad age range of clients since it is suitable for preschool children (from 6.5 to 7 years) to adults.

The CSD multidisciplinary and multidimensional team approach in diagnostics and treatment makes it possible to identify nearly all concomitant stuttering problems and to address stuttering in a holistic fashion. Another advantage is that we combine different treatment formats. A combination of individual and group, as well as residential and outpatient treatment obtain the best outcomes for each client. Each of these treatment formats has a different purpose. The CSD also has rigorous follow-up procedures for the purpose of avoiding relapse or minimising it in case it occurs. Members of the client's family, their friends, teachers and colleagues are included in the therapy. This has the effect of educating them about stuttering and helps them to see it in a more positive way. They can then be a source of support to the client.

Treatment is well structured and easy to apply once a person is familiar with it. Additionally, an advantage of CSD is that no technical equipment is necessary.

Disadvantages

A disadvantage of CSD is that it requires a great deal of commitment from the client, therefore, some do not return after initial diagnostics and some do not complete the treatment (Brajović and Brajović, 1976, 1981). Some drop out after Phase I or during Phase II (Jelčić Jakšić et al., 2003); sometimes they will return several months or years later. The reason for dropouts is that some clients may find the programme too demanding due to its long-term commitment and the effort needed to change themselves. We also find that because speech therapy is covered by health insurance in Serbia, some clients tend to prolong their treatment for longer than is necessary. It is also the case that the treatment relies heavily on individual therapists within the team, which has some disadvantages (Plexico et al., 2010). Finally, we do not have any long-term outcome data for CSD as yet.

Conclusions and future directions

Although the data are from preliminary file audits, there are reasons to believe that the CSD method may be successful in providing a holistic framework for stuttering treatment, based on a holistic view of humans. It is well organised but is also flexible enough to be used for treating a broad spectrum of clients, from preschool children to adults. It combines individual, group, outpatient and residential settings for clients and families, and encourages clients to be their own therapists. The approach has existed for over 40 years and, arguably, has proven its value over that period. We are satisfied with the results so far, but there is always room for improvement and we plan to implement changes to achieve this.

For the future we plan to introduce self-help group into Phase III of the programme with the goal of making clients self-reliant earlier. We also need to improve our treatment gains for stress caused by listener reaction; this dimension currently shows the least improvement of our three reported variables. As a part of the future development of the treatment, we plan to integrate feedback from clients, their families and our colleagues, in the interests of improving the treatment. And finally, we recognise that in the future we need to pay closer attention to evaluating treatment outcomes.

Discussion

Sheena Reilly
The first thing we would like to have is a description of what time tracking is. Our group had about five different definitions of what it might be, so could you tell us what you mean by time tracking?

Jelena Tadić

I never actually defined it, but time tracking is essential if you are going to speak. You need to know how long what you are about to say is, so you can incorporate how much air you need in order to monitor the passing of time while you are speaking. So the video we showed[2] was a client who first had the goal of singing correctly for a certain amount of time. When a certain amount of time passed without a clock she had to say how long it was, and ask herself, 'Could I really do what I planned in that amount of time?' Because people have the feeling that they have to finish the task and they often speed up. It's the same for me here, I'm not very good at the moment, I am speeding up, but do I really need to? I can allow myself time to say it slowly.

Sheena Reilly

So you would preset a time for a task and then the client would do the task and then reflect on whether the client allowed enough time. Is that the essence of it?

Jelena Tadić

Yes, I believe it is.

Ann Packman

And to follow up on that, what do you mean by sensory integration?

Jelena Tadić

Throughout therapy, clients are taught gradually to raise awareness and work on development of many aspects of sensory skills, such as listening, voicing, fine motor movements, kinaesthetic feedback, a sense of rhythm and time. This is what is meant by sensory integration. By enhancing their ability to focus on those skills, clients learn to gain control over their speech and react appropriately in speech situations.

Ann Packman

We had some discussion about how your treatments might differ for the very young child compared to the adults. Would you do fluency shaping with young children?

Jelena Tadić

For the very young we do something else. CSD is for preschoolers who are already aware of their stuttering, who already have had some negative experiences with it, who are willing to participate and willing to put in some effort. We make it a bit more fun and of course, we do not engage the reading and writing side of the programme until the children are fluent in reading and writing. What I do notice is that when they start to read, they do not stutter much on reading. When stuttering while reading occurs, that is a good time to incorporate reading exercises, introducing speech exercises into reading, so we are practically following the child's reading development practically. We also work with parents on their own attitudes towards stuttering and also their

---

[2] The presenters showed a video of a client demonstrating this time tracking procedure.

attitudes towards their child. Sometimes family therapy is needed to deal with such matters. If the child has additional speech and language problems we will also try to remediate those and to work on them too, maybe not directly on articulation but definitely on the oral motor skills that are helpful, I think, both for articulation and also awareness of articulatory movements. During all this we try to make it fun by telling stories and playing games to engage the children.

Joseph Attanasio

Could we have further clarification on the differences between treatment for adults and the preschoolers? For the preschoolers, is it the goal to eliminate or nearly eliminate the stuttering? Is the goal that the treatment is durable for children? Or as for adults, is vigilance needed to prevent relapse? Would you expect the children to come back when they are adults?

Jelena Tadić

Mostly we don't expect them to come back and mostly they do not come back if they went through the whole programme. It depends not only on the child but, as I said, on the parents and the family as well. With the Lidcombe Program you also find that the family is very important for maintaining fluency. But, yes, the goal would be to achieve fluency, maybe not perfect fluency but close to it and also to achieve positive attitudes, to help ensure there are no negative feelings about stuttering in either children or parents. If you achieve that, then very often you can see fluency getting better and better in time as they use the recipe for what to do as part of their daily routine. For example, 'now let's do a bit of reading', 'now let's do a bit of something else'. That makes it less like therapy and more like just a part of their daily lives.

Sheena Reilly

Do you have criteria for moving from each phase of the treatment to the next?

Jelena Tadić

We do have some general criteria that can be adjusted to individual needs and abilities of the client. Going from Phase I into Phase II we do not expect transfer to other speaking situations. We expect that during Phase III. During Phase I-II we require clients to master the applied techniques for breathing and speech, so they are ready for the Phase III group work. We do not see change dramatically overnight, but then if you allow yourself the time to assimilate it all then there is a high probability of success.

Ann Packman

You said that you would like to gather more data and perhaps do a clinical trial. It is such a comprehensive programme, so what would you consider the primary outcome measures?

Jelena Tadić

The goal of the programme is reduced stuttering together with improved satisfaction in speech situations. Some will drop out of the programme once they feel good and their residual stuttering does not interfere with their life. So we would need both measures of fluency and client satisfaction. We would need separate measures for preschoolers because we would have to include parental attitudes.

Joseph Attanasio

Could you describe or identify the team members and what their responsibilities are?

Jelena Tadić

It is always a speech pathologist and psychologist, and in our institute we have a neurologist, a paediatrician and a physiotherapist. Also, hearing screening is conducted, as well as intellectual testing for all clients. There will also be personality testing if recommended jointly by a psychologist and a speech pathologist. In some cases, clients will need to be referred to a psychiatrist for additional help. The neurologist will also screen for neurological problems that seem to be interfering with the treatment.

Joseph Attanasio

Does every client go through that battery of tests?

Jelena Tadić

Every client, yes.

Sheena Reilly

Can you expand on your relaxation procedures?

Jelena Tadić

It is guided by clients' Subjective Units of Distress scores from 0 to 100. During relaxation, the first instruction is of course relaxation, followed by imagining a safe place and then from that safe place imagining going into speech situations that you choose. We usually choose a situation to start that has a Subjective Units of Distress score between 40 and 50, because 30 does not interfere really with everyday life. When clients can remain in a relaxed state while imagining the situation, we begin role-play in that situation. After a role-play with the clinician, the client and patient together with the clients will role-play that scenario. And then the rest of group will reflect on what they saw. 'Were you self-confident or not?' 'Okay, you were stuttering but you seemed to be very self-confident' and so on.

Sheena Reilly

So that is group feedback?

Jelena Tadić

Yes.

Ann Packman

You mentioned bringing the clients consciously back to how they were before they were stuttering. What did you mean by that?

Jelena Tadić

We try to have our clients remember what it was like before they started to stutter. Many of our clients do remember. They may say, 'I started to stutter when I was five or six or when I started school'. Some normal behaviours and abilities were already developed, because of the normal processes of child development. Bringing them back into conscious memory provides a focus to speak as before.

Joseph Attanasio
How long does this treatment take?

Jelena Tadić
The average treatment time is approximately 12 months, excluding maintenance and follow-up. Not everyone can come for the period of residential treatment because of work and other obligations, and if that is the case then treatment generally takes longer. Perhaps measurement of treatment time is something that we need for our future work.

Ann Packman
It has been obvious over the last few days how much funding determines what treatment we can give. Does your government fund this treatment, or do people have to pay privately?

Jelena Tadić
People usually do not pay privately. There is no charge for those who pay health insurance. However, it appears as if in the future only a specific number of treatment sessions will be available, to cut out the problem I mentioned of clients prolonging treatments unnecessarily

Ann Packman
So does everyone pay health insurance?

Jelena Tadić
Yes, 99% of Serbians.

References

Ambrose, N. G. (2008) Possible genetic factors in subtypes of stuttering. 1st European Symposium on Fluency Disorders. Lessius University College, Antwerp, Belgium; April.

Archibald, L., & De Nil, L. F. (1999) The relationship between stuttering severity and kinesthetic acuity for jaw movements in adults who stutter. *Journal of Fluency Disorders, 24*, 25-42.

Beck, A. T. (1975) *Cognitive Therapy and the Emotional Disorders*. New York: International Universities Press Inc.

Brajović, C., & Brajović, Lj. (1976) *Rehabilitacija Poremećaja Funkcije Govora*. Beograd, Republika Srbija: Naučna knjiga.

Brajović, C., & Brajović, Lj. (1981) *Rehabilitacija Poremecaja Funkcije Govora*. Beograd, Republika Srbija: Naučna knjiga.

Brajović, Lj., Popović, L., & Šešum, M. (2010) *Monografija Zavoda za Psihofiziološke Poremećaje, i Govornu Patologiju "Profesor Dr Cvetko Brajović"*. Beograd, Republika Srbija: Narodna biblioteka Srbije.

De Nil, L. F., Kroll, R. M., & Houle, S. (2001) Functional neuroimaging of cerebellar activation during single word reading and verb generation in stuttering and nonstuttering adults. *Neuroscience Letters, 302*, 77-80.

Dobrota-Davidović, N., Petrovic-Lazic, M., Šoster, D., & Jovanovic-Simic, N. (2007) Voice analysis of person who stutter. 2nd Congress of Slovenian Logopedists with international participation: The quality of Slovenian logopedia in Europe, Proceedings, Maribor, Slovenia; pp. 158-160.

Eggers, K., De Nil, L. F., & Van den Berg, B. R. H. (2010) Temperament dimensions in stuttering and typically developing children. *Journal of Fluency Disorders*, 35, 355-372.

Fibiger, S., Peters, H. F. M., Euler, H. A., & Neumann, K. (2008) Health and human services for persons who stutter and education of logopedists in East-European countries. *Journal of Fluency Disorders*, 33, 66-71.

Guitar, B. (2006) *Stuttering: An Integrated Approach to Its Nature and Treatment* (3rd ed.). Baltimore, MD: Lippincott Williams and Wilkins.

Jelčić, S. (1992) Svjesna sinteza razvoja u terapiji poremećaja ritma i tempa govora. In: F. Ibrahimpašić & S. Jelčic (Eds.), *Govorna Komunikacija*. Zagreb, Croatia: Zavod Za Zaštitu Zdravlja Grada Zagreba i Naklada Slap.

Jelčić Jakšić, S. (2002) My story: From group sessions to national association, Međunarodni naučni skup "Dani Zavoda". *Zbornik Rezimea* (pp. 56-57). Beograd, Republika Srbija.

Jelčić Jakšić, S., Lasan, M., Rowley, D., & Sardelić, S. (2002) An evaluation of the use SSR method in the Centre for Speech disorders in Zagreb, Međunarodni naučni skup "Dani Zavoda". *Zbornik Rezimea* (pp. 44-45). Beograd, Republika Srbija.

Jelčić Jakšić, S., Lasan, M., & Rowley, D. (2003) The relationship between stuttering severity and willingness to complete therapy. Proceedings of the 1st Congress of Slovenian Speech and Language Pathologists with international participation: Speech and Language Therapy for All Stages of Life, Bled, Slovenija; pp. 108-111.

Namasivayam, A. K., & van Lieshout, P. (2008) Investigating speech motor practice and learning in people who stutter. *Journal of Fluency Disorders*, 33, 32-51.

Plexico, L. W., Manning, W. H., & DiLollo, A. (2010) Client perceptions of effective and ineffective therapeutic alliances during treatment for stuttering. *Journal of Fluency Disorders*, 35, 333-354.

Podbrežnik, V., & Čepelnik, J. (2002) With Will to Demosthenes by the Method of Conscious Synthesis of Development and Method VLAJA, Međunarodni naučni skup "Dani Zavoda", *Zbornik Rezimea* (pp. 42-43). Beograd, Republika Srbija.

Podbrežnik, V., & Čepelnik, J. (2010) The method of conscious synthesis of development. In: *Monografija Zavoda za Psihofiziološke Poremećaje i Govornu Patologiju "Profesor Dr Cvetko Brajović"* (pp. 179-197). Beograd, Republika Srbija: Narodna biblioteka Srbije.

Radonjić, J. (1982) Sistematska desenzitizacija kao metod redukcije anksioznosti u terapiji mucanja, Magistarski rad, Beograd, Republika Srbija.

Simić-Ružić, B., & Jovanović, A. (2008) Family characteristics of stuttering children. *Srpski Arhiv za Celokupno Lekarstvo*, 136(11-12), 629-634.

Šoster, D. (2003) Reduction of anxiety during the stationary group treatment of adult stutterers. Proceedings of the 1st Congress of Slovenian Speech and Language Pathologists with international participation: Speech and Language Therapy for all Stages of Life, Bled, Slovenia; pp. 112-115.

Šoster, D., Dobrota-Davidović, N., & Tadić, J. (2007) Reduction of subjective distress caused by co-speakers reactions actived during stationary group treatment of adult stutterers. 2nd Congress of Slovenian logopedists with international participation "The quality of Slovenian logopedia in Europe", Proceedings, Maribor, Slovenia; pp.135-137.

Tadić, J., Šoster, D., & Dobrota-Davidović, N. (2009) Oral apraxia and stuttering. Istraživanja u specijalnoj edukaciji i rehabilitaciji, Univerzitet u Beogradu - Fakultet za specijalnu edukaciju i rehabilitaciju; pp.79-88.

Tadić, J., Šoster, D., Dobrota-Davidović, N., & Jovanovic-Simic, N. (2010) Subjective distress caused by co-speakers' reactions - reduction during stationary group treatment. *Journal of Special Education and Rehabilitation*, *11* (1-2), 39-52.

Van Riper, C. (1973) *The Treatment of Stuttering*. Englewood Cliffs, NJ: Prentice-Hall.

Watkins, K. E., Smith, S. M., Davis, S., & Howell, P. (2008) Structural and functional abnormalities of the motor system in developmental stuttering. *Brain*, *131*(1), 50-59.

Wolpe, J. (1958) *Psychotherapy by Reciprocal Inhibition*. Stanford, CA: Stanford University Press.

Wolpe, J. (1969) *The Practice of Behavior Therapy*. New York: Pergamon Press.

Chapter 17

The Gradual Increase in Length and Complexity of Utterance Program

Bruce Ryan

California State University, Long Beach, Long Beach, CA, USA

Overview

The Gradual Increase in Length and Complexity of Utterance (GILCU) pro-gramme is a programmed operant treatment for those who stutter of all ages. As an operant treatment, the intention is for its treatment procedures to be outlined in a clear and replicable fashion. Its outcomes are expressed in terms of objective pre-treatment and post-treatment stuttered words per minute (SWM) and the duration of treatment in hours. Normal speech fluency is defined as less than 3.0 SWM. Control speakers have been shown to have a mean SWM of 1.2 (SD $=$ 0.7) (Ryan, 2001a). During treatment, no attention is ever paid to secondary stuttering characteristics or other cognitive–emotive aspects of stuttering. The focus of GILCU is normal fluent speech.

The learning format of GILCU is drawn from operant conditioning principles (Skinner, 1953). These embrace: (1) objective, observable behaviour; (2) small steps from easy to difficult; and (3) immediate consequences for each desired (fluent) behaviour and undesired (stuttering) behaviour. The core of this treat-ment programme is systematic progression from small to large behavioural steps that are immediately reinforced or punished, leading to an end-goal re-sponse of normal fluency. The GILCU programme comprises an Establishment programme, followed by out-of-clinic Transfer and Maintenance programmes, which are employed after GILCU is completed (Ryan, 2001a).

The GILCU Establishment programme contains 54 regular steps, and 59 branch steps if failure occurs on any regular step. GILCU starts with the client reading one word through one sentence fluently for up to 30 seconds, through 5 minutes of fluent reading in 18 steps. The sequence is then repeated with monologue, and then conversation. Home practice is begun after completion

The Science and Practice of Stuttering Treatment: A Symposium, First Edition. Edited by Suzana Jelčić Jakšić and Mark Onslow.
© 2012 John Wiley & Sons, Ltd. Published 2012 by John Wiley & Sons, Ltd.

of each mode. The treatment targets are stuttered words or syllables and fluent words or syllables. Stuttered words or syllables are consequated by the clinician who says, 'Stop', and when the client pauses, says, 'Speak fluently'. Fluent responses are followed by 'Good'. There is very slight revision of GILCU in the latest Ryan and Ryan (2005) version[1], mostly in record keeping and amount of testing time.

There are presently two versions of the original Transfer programme: one in Ryan and Van Kirk (1978) and Ryan (2001a) composed of nine series and 54 steps. The series include home, audience and telephone speaking situations. The second version, Ryan and Ryan (2005), is for school-age children and is a simplified form of the original, with only five series of three to five steps each.

For preschool children, there is a simplified version of GILCU that involves no reading and reduced duration of assessments, and simplified Transfer and Maintenance programmes (Ryan, 2001a).

Theoretical basis

A detailed discussion of the theoretical basis of the programme is presented in Ryan (1979). Stuttered speech is a motor response that is learned through operant conditioning (Shames and Sherrick, 1963), but may also have a physiological brain processing component underpinning it. Moore (1984, 1993) published findings suggesting that hemispheric processing may best explain the neurophysiological underpinnings of stuttering. I have observed some preschool stuttering children change from demonstrating severe to no stuttering over a matter of few days, weeks or months with no treatment or environmental change. Hemispheric processing could explain this rapid, unassisted, extensive change. Simply put, the left hemisphere is better suited than the right for managing speech fluency. For some unknown reason, 1–3% of 2–5-year-old children 'accidentally' start processing speech fluency on the right instead of the left hemisphere. This results in stuttering. At least 70% of these stuttering children, using their own devices, transfer back to the left hemisphere before or by the time they are 7 years old, and speak normally fluently.

Demonstrated value

Ryan (2001a) presented an overview of 208 participants in outcome studies, ranging in age from 4 to 45 years. Data for 61 of these participants were previously unpublished. The two basic, within-clinic procedures for collecting data were the Fluency Interview, which included 10 different speaking tasks including reading and telephone, and the Criterion Test, which involved 2–5 minutes each of reading, monologue and conversation (Ryan, 2001a). The Fluency Interview was used to select participants who were over 3.0 SWM for treatment. The Criterion Test is used to enter the GILCU and to pass

[1]Readers can obtain a copy of this author published manuscript by contacting the author at bpryan@csulb.edu.

through the Establishment, Transfer and Maintenance programmes using a criterion of 0.5 SWM. We commonly use and report both for pre-treatment and post-treatment results.

Ryan (2001a) reported a mean Pre-establishment SWM score of 9.2 (range 5.9–10.4) and a mean Post-establishment score of 0.2 SWM (range 0.2–2.5). Corresponding improvements of speech rate in words spoken per minute were reported from a mean of 92.4 Pre-establishment to 109.2 Post-establishment. The mean treatment time reported for these effects in Ryan (2001a), in terms of 'talk time', was 8.1 hours, with a range of 5–7 hours. Ryan notes that this would equate to around double the treatment time in clinical hours. Ryan (1981) presented follow-up data for nine school-age children, mean age 11.1 years (range 7–16 years) who received treatment within their school environment. The mean follow-up period was 12.5 months (range 7–20 months). Mean Pre-establishment SWM was 6.5 (range 3.6–10.2) and the mean follow-up SWM was 0.6 (range 0–1.2).

Early intervention for preschoolers is thought by many to be desirable, although the known 70% natural recovery rate of this population (Yairi and Ambrose, 2005) must be controlled for in client selection, lest we divert attention from those who will not recover to treat those who will. Therefore, another treatment variation for preschoolers is extended base rate observation for at least three to four times every 3–5 months, for at least 9–15 months, to determine stability of the stuttering response. If the stuttering is naturally decreasing, the child is on the recovery path and therapy should be withheld, with extended base rate continued until the child shows stability of under 3.0 SWM for a second year. If the rate is stable or increasing during that first observation year, then the child should be offered treatment of GILCU or the Lidcombe Program (see Chapter 4). After several more years of follow-up of both groups, this procedure proved to be 95% accurate in selecting persistent stuttering clients for treatment. Figure 17.1 presents some results about this

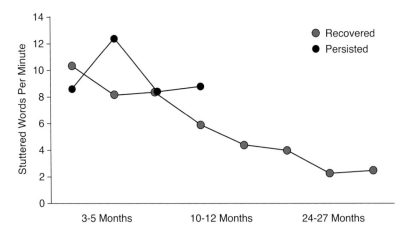

Figure 17.1 Stuttered words per minute scores over 2 years for a group of persisting and naturally recovering preschool children. (Reprinted from Ryan (2001b), with permission from Elsevier.)

topic from Ryan (2001b), showing two groups of preschool stuttering children aged 2–5 years. One group ($N = 7$) persisted and one group ($N = 15$) naturally recovered. This provided a natural recovery rate of 68%, which is broadly consistent with the Yairi and Ambrose (2005) results. Based on these results, we have used the extended base rate procedure to select persisted clients for treatment. In short, we have very little GILCU data with preschoolers because most recovered naturally, and/or we also focused on doing Phase I trials on other independent variables like interruption or experimental programmes like 'slow' talk with children who did not recover. In short, I have not used the preschool version of the GILCU programme very much, only reporting on one 4-year-old child in Ryan (2001a).

Advantages and disadvantages

Advantages

The GILCU Establishment programme is easy to administer to clients and to teach to student clinicians. The programme has been conducted successfully by many different trained clinicians (Ryan, 1981, 2001a). It requires only that the clinician be able to accurately and consistently identify stuttered words and/or syllables and provide appropriate consequences and the client to be able to speak fluently for gradually longer and longer utterances or time periods, starting with one word up to sentences, and then 1 minute up to 5 minutes of talking.

This programme has been successful in the schools, partly because in the American school system the students and their parents are easily available, especially for transfer and maintenance. The Individuals with Disabilities Education Act of 1975 is a US federal law[2] that mandates individual educational programmes as needed. The Act requires that at least one parent comes to the school to develop and participate in any treatment programme planning and execution for any 3–21-year-old person who has been identified with a special problem, including stuttering. GILCU has been used in the United Kingdom (Rustin et al., 1987). Additionally, GILCU has been used successfully in several countries in a non-English language: Mandarin (Ryan, 1998) and German (Scheppe and Jehle, 1985).

Disadvantages

My clinical experience and research has shown that a weakness of GILCU is that it is less effective with more severe clients, particularly teenagers or adults (Ryan and Ryan, 1983, 1995). In my view, clients must 'find' their own way to speak fluently and some with severe stuttering cannot achieve that. For those few failure clients with GILCU, we have then used the DAF-Prolongation Establishment programme (Ryan, 2001a), or we have pre-sorted

[2]http://en.wikipedia.org/wiki/United_States_federal_law.

the severe clients into DAF-prolongation programmes (Rustin et al., 1987). Another potential disadvantage of GILCU is that some clinicians have trouble identifying and consequating stuttering even after training. It is also the case that transfer is difficult for some clinicians to arrange in private practice settings.

It is not a disadvantage of GILCU, but a disadvantage for people who stutter, that GILCU is not used by the speech pathology profession. In my opinion, based on examination of the literature and the American Speech-Language-Hearing website, GILCU is not widely known nor recognised nor practiced in our profession by people who treat stuttering. It is not taught in our university professional preparation programmes nor adequately cited with data in our modern speech-language pathology textbooks.

Conclusions and future directions

Evaluation of the GILCU programme shows that normal, permanent speech fluency is an attainable goal for people who stutter of all ages. After over 40 years of evidence-based practice and clinical research on over 200 clients using GILCU or a variation, to establish fluent speech, I believe GILCU has been shown to be a powerful, effective, easy to use and easy to teach procedure for helping people who stutter of all ages to speak fluently. The new short-ened version is designed especially for school-age children for use by public school clinicians (Ryan and Ryan, 2005). This shortened version is still us-able for adults with additional transfer procedures drawn from Ryan (2001a). This programme should be taught and practiced in every university training programme and be in the therapy repertoire of every speech-language pathol-ogist who works with people who stutter. Our past research during which we gave students only the self-instructional materials and a week to study them before they went into treatment with a client, revealed that they were able to self-learn the programme in hours and conduct it out well with their clients, with only a few problems (Ryan and McMicken, 2007).

Discussion

Ann Packman

We were wondering what is meant by the statement that the procedures lead to 'normal fluency'? How do you know that stutter-free speech is normally fluent speech?

Bruce Ryan

We refer to our data gathered from the Fluency Interview given to over 400 normally fluent people, male and female speakers aged 3-63, as judged by themselves and people who knew them (Ryan, 2001a). We considered (1) type of stuttered word, such as whole- and part-word repetition, prolongation and struggle, (2) rate of stuttered words and (3) speaking rate. We assume normal fluency, if, post-treatment, our stuttering clients speak within one SD either above or below each of the means of these three parameters for normally fluent speakers of varying ages with no struggle. Rarely did our normally fluent speakers demonstrate struggle. Finally, our clients must sound normally fluent to us by casual observation or formal naturalness ratings (Ryan, 2001a).

Ann Packman

This all raises the issue that it seems paradoxical that normal speech can contain stuttering. What do you say to that?

Bruce Ryan

No, not at all. One may stutter occasionally and not be a stutterer. For example, the stuttered utterances of 'c-car' or 'car-car' or 'caaar' can and are spoken by almost all normally fluent speakers as well as stutterers. This is not true for struggle. The difference is the rate of occurrence. If the speaker emits above 3% of words spoken, or 1.5 percent syllables stuttered (%SS; Ryan, 2001a), the speaker is considered to be a stutterer by both lay people and most speech professionals. Few normally fluent speakers are 100% fluent, according to our numerous hours of audiotape of normally fluent speakers. These cut-offs have been very functional both to select clients and to decide whether treated clients have reached normal fluency. Basic research was done on this point by Wendell Johnson in the 1940s and many speech-language pathologists have built their classification systems on his work, as have I.

Ann Packman

Can you elaborate on which of your data sets support your statement that the programme has been extremely effective in the American school system.

Bruce Ryan

The best data sets for GILCU in the public schools are to be found in Ryan (2001a) and Ryan and Ryan (1983, 1995). I was motivated to study operant programmes, like GILCU, in the public schools, because of the large number of stuttering children found in the public schools in America. We researched treatment programmes that were developed by us, but conducted by public school clinicians while carrying out their regular duties with their other regular clients in their respective public schools. These clinicians were trained and supervised by us to control for administration validity. Further, Barbara Ryan has worked in the public schools of Southern California for the past 33 years and has collected extensive, but as yet unpublished data, using GILCU with her public school stuttering clients. She has reported to me that she has seldom failed to establish fluent, normal speech. Follow-up, conducted by her, indicated that the children had remained fluent.

Ann Packman

Can you give us more details about how you collected the outcome measures obtained for the studies you overviewed?

Bruce Ryan

The Fluency Interview and Criterion Tests were done with the clinician in the clinic room, pre-establishment, post-establishment, post-transfer, post-maintenance and at follow-up. We also measured clients' stuttering during all transfer steps, such as speaking in the classroom or at work, and at follow-up. The number of steps varied with the client's age. Most often, in the first transfer activities, the clinician was there and counted and recorded stuttered words. In some of the latter Transfer programme steps, depending on age and ability, the client self-recorded on a small tape recorder, or simply reported stuttered words. These outside measures served to check the client's speech in the natural environment. We compared these to our in-clinic measures and found them quite comparable. We also asked for self-reports from the client or client's parents about the client's stuttering, which generally reflected the improvement shown in the SWM measures.

Joseph Attanasio

Your programme requires that clinicians can accurately and consistently identify stuttered words and syllables. Is there evidence available for the accuracy and consistency of those clinician judgments? Certainly, other researchers have found this to be a problem.

Bruce Ryan

It is a problem. We all need to accurately identify and count stuttering events, if we are to conduct operant conditioning programmes that require appropriate, immediate consequences for the undesired responses of stuttered syllables and words and the desired responses of fluent syllables and words. We noted the problem in Ryan and Ryan (1983). To develop a classification system, I used basically the Johnson (1961) dual categories of normal disfluencies: interjections, revision, incomplete phrases, phrase repetitions, pauses and stuttered disfluencies, whole- and part-word repetitions, prolongations and struggle disfluencies (Ryan, 1974). Later, I modified this system to break down the categories of whole- and part- word repetition each into single and multiple repetitions after Yairi and Ambrose (2005) for my research with preschool children (Ryan, 2001a). Normal fluency would be defined as the absence or low rate (< 3.0 SWM) of stuttered disfluencies. I have always used and taught a classification system with the belief that such a system aided the identifier in counting accuracy, more of a match-to-sample or sort task rather than a simple identification of behaviours like 'unambiguous stuttering'. Clinician observers were trained on this system to a high degree of accuracy using audio- and video-recorded samples (e.g. Ryan, 2001a; Ryan and Van Kirk, 1974). In addition, I used numerous inter- and intra-reliability procedures, commonly percentage agreement of simple counts between two or more observer clinicians. In my research with preschoolers, we also made scripts of our conversations with subjects and did point-to-point counts in our determination of reliability. We have striven for and usually achieved better than 90% agreement, or did more training, if we did not. The answer to your question is that there is an abundance of evidence of reliability measures in my research and that of others that clinicians can achieve high accuracy of identifying and counting with or without using the elaborate procedures of a classification system and audio-video training that I did.

Joseph Attanasio

Given that the programme has been in use for 40 years, we were wondering why randomised controlled trials have not been done.

Bruce Ryan

The programme appeared to be running well, in my purview, and according to our research. See the results of eight studies that I reported previously. Also, one could describe our research reported in Ryan and Ryan (1983, 1995) as a stratified random sampling design, advanced for the time of data collection during 1972-1974. Participants in these two studies were children who were 6 years of age or older. Almost all were past the age of spontaneous recovery, were able to read and had a high probability of persistence. My wife, Barbara Ryan has run the programme very successfully in the public schools from 1978 to 2011. She often said that she never failed to help a school-age stuttering child become normally fluent. Unfortunately, she has not been able to share these data because of local school privacy of information policy. We eventually shortened the programme (Ryan and Ryan, 2005) and still she has achieved equal success using it primarily with school-age children. We have run the original GILCU (Ryan, 2001a) in my University clinic since 1978, then have tested the self-instructional form of the programme for 5 years with similar positive results (Ryan and McMicken, 2007).

Joseph Attanasio

Given the evidence in support of the Lidcombe Program for early stuttering and the Camperdown Program for adolescents and adults, both of which are non-programmed treatments, what are the arguments in favour of a highly structured and programmed approach such as GILCU?

Bruce Ryan

The major value of tight structure, as in the GILCU programme, is accuracy of replication, important both for scientific investigation and effectiveness. As I discuss in Ryan (2001a), careful examination of the Lidcombe Program reveals that it may have more structure and be more programmed than the authors realise. As an update, I recently re-read both the current guides for the Camperdown Program and the Lidcombe Program. I noted a great amount of detail in these latest instructional manuals, including score sheets and rating scale data sheets. True, there were few criterion levels (save for %SS levels for passing some treatment phases, but still, in my opinion, these manuals, and the programmes they describe, very closely approximate at least 'train loosely' (Stokes and Baer, 1977) programmed instruction. I would speculate that in actual practice, the Lidcombe Program and the Camperdown Program are not that much different in basic structure and operant logic from the GILCU programme; they both use observable behaviour, small, sequential steps towards a goal of reduced or no unambiguous stuttering and appropriate consequences for desired and undesired behaviour.

Joseph Attanasio

There are several components to your very meticulous response, but I would like to follow-up on what seems to be your relevant point. That is, your statement that the only advantage you can see for tight programming is the accuracy of replication or treatment integrity, also called treatment fidelity. Might the case be the opposite of what you suggest? That is, the more tightly programmed the treatment, the more likely it might be that clinicians and researchers would err in following treatment steps in the manner those steps are prescribed and, at the same time, the less likely would treatment take advantage of the individual ways in which clients successfully respond to treatment and of the ways in which clinicians (or parents, in the case of Lidcombe) successfully adapt treatment to fit the needs and responses of clients? In short, might tight programming be unnecessarily rigid and prone to error?

Bruce Ryan

Anything is possible, but I thought we were in the context of science, not speculation. I think structure and clarity of procedures are important assets of programmed instruction, which lead to replication, an important facet of science itself. Our observations have been that clinicians do adapt the GILCU programme regardless of what they have been taught and how clearly the programme is described (Ryan and Ryan, 1983, 1995). Further, we have seen what they do 'intuitively' has often been to the detriment of the efficacy of the programme (Ryan, 2001a). While supervising, we have often had to say, 'Stick to the programme!' Programmes based on operant conditioning principles use these principles to solve the problems that arise during the construction and testing of the programme, not people's instinctive or intuitive problem-solving abilities. For example, when we worried about the possibility that teenagers might not want to show up for treatment or do their home practice, we did not leave it to their parents or school clinicians or the teens themselves to intuitively solve the problem; we increased the reinforcement system, which solved the problem. When I worried about accidentally treating preschool children who might spontaneously recover, I did not elect to treat them all, instead we studied preschool stuttering children, giving them no therapy until the extended baseline trend of their stuttering behaviour over a year from the first observation was found to predict natural recovery or persistence (Ryan, 2001b).

Finally, how would one scientifically measure or control for the intuitive contributions made to the success of any treatment programme? If client, clinician and parent intuition are part of the programme, then there would be as many different programmes as there were clients, clinicians, and parents, along with their various intuitive behaviours.

References

Johnson, W. (1961) Measurements of oral reading and speaking rate and disfluency of adult male and female stutterers and nonstutterers. *Journal of Speech and Hearing Disorders. Monograph Supplement*(No. 7), 1-20.

Moore, W. (1984) Central nervous system characteristics of stutterers. In: R. Curlee & W. Perkins (Eds.), *Nature and Treatment of Stuttering: New Directions* (pp. 49-72). San Diego, CA: College-Hill.

Moore, W. (1993) Hemispheric processing research: past, present, and future. In: E. Boberg (Ed.), *Neuropsychology of Stuttering* (pp. 39-72). Edmonton, Alberta, Canada: University of Alberta Press.

Rustin, L., Ryan, B., & Ryan, B. (1987) Use of the Monterey programmed stuttering treatment in Great Britain. *British Journal of Disorders of Communication, 22*, 151-162.

Ryan, B. (1974) *Programmed Stuttering Therapy for Children and Adults*. Springfield, IL: CC Thomas.

Ryan, B. (1979) Stuttering treatment in a framework of operant conditioning. In: H. Gregory (Ed.), *Controversies About Stuttering Treatment* (pp. 129-144). Baltimore, MD: University Park Press.

Ryan, B. (1981) Maintenance programs in progress-II. In: E. Boberg (Ed.), *Maintenance of Fluency* (pp. 113-146). New York: Elsevier North Holland Inc.

Ryan, B. (1998) The use of the Monterey Fluency Program in Hong Kong (Abstract). Paper presented at the first Asia-Pacific Speech, Language, and Hearing Conference. Hong Kong. *Asia Pacific Journal of Speech, Language, and Hearing, 3*, 164-165.

Ryan, B. (2001a) *Programmed Stuttering Therapy for Children and Adults* (2nd ed.). Springfield, IL: Charles C. Thomas.

Ryan, B. (2001b) A longitudinal study of the articulation, language, rate, and fluency of 22 preschool children. *Journal of Fluency Disorders, 26*, 107-127.

Ryan, B., & McMicken, B. (2007) Evidence-based practice in universities: teaching students an evidence-based treatment. Research, treatment, and self-help in fluency disorders: new horizons. Proceedings of the Fifth World Congress on Fluency Disorders. The International Fluency Association; pp. 298-303.

Ryan, B., & Ryan, B. V. (1983) Programmed stuttering therapy for children: comparison of four establishment programs. *Journal of Fluency Disorders, 8*, 291-321.

Ryan, B., & Ryan, B. V. (1995) Programmed stuttering therapy for children: comparison of two establishment programs, through transfer, maintenance, and follow-up. *Journal of Speech and Hearing Research, 38*, 61-75.

Ryan, B., & Van Kirk, B. (1974) The establishment, transfer, and maintenance of fluent speech in 50 stutterers using delayed auditory feedback and operant procedures. *Journal of Speech and Hearing Disorders, 39*, 3-10.

Ryan, B., & Van Kirk, B. (1978) *Monterey Fluency Program*. Palo Alto, CA: Monterey Learning Systems.

Ryan, B. V., & Ryan, B. P. (2005) *The Ryan fluency program workbook*. Long Beach, CA: Authors.

Scheppe, D., & Jehle, P. (1985) Das Monterey-Sprechtraining Program in der praxis. *Die Sprachheilarbeit, 30*(5), 217-224.

Shames, G., & Sherrick, C. (1963) A discussion of nonfluency and stuttering as operant behavior. *Journal of Speech and Hearing Disorders, 28*, 3-18.

Skinner, B. F. (1953) *Science and Human Behavior*. New York: Macmillan.

Stokes, T., & Baer, D. (1977) An implicit technology of generalization. *Journal of Applied Behavioral Analysis, 10*, 349-367.

Yairi, E., & Ambrose, N. (2005) *Early Childhood Stuttering: For Clinicians by Clinicians*. Austin, TX: Pro-Ed.

Chapter 18

Innovations, Watersheds and Gold Standards: Concluding Symposium Reflections

Mark Onslow

The University of Sydney, Sydney, Australia

Innovation at last

On reflection after this extensive event, one feature more than all others comes to mind. Naturally enough, regardless of whether we are clinicians or researchers, or both, we are inevitably to some extent positioned by the intellectual and scientific climates of our background professional literature. Those of us with an English-speaking background are informed mostly by the English language literature, and the literature of other languages during the course of our professional lives is fundamentally inaccessible – Serbian and Italian, in the case of this Symposium. Conversely, those with non-English backgrounds would not have routine access to the English language professional literature. Although, to their credit, the reference lists of our Italian and Serbian delegates show that they were far more influenced by the English language literature in the formulation of their treatment procedures than were the English-speaking delegates influenced by the output of European literature.

One message the Convenors took home from the symposium is the strong benefit of combining representatives from diverse professional backgrounds to share their ideas at such a forum. As stated in the preface, another iteration of the symposium is planned. That likely will occur during 2013, but will not be about a clinical topic. However, the plan is for the symposium to be a 3-yearly event, and eventually, we will cycle back to a clinical theme. At which time we would hope to redress the imbalance that we saw during 2010 and ensure that clinical presentations at such a future event are more evenly balanced between European and non-European input.

Not surprisingly then, our Serbian and Italian colleagues presented the most refreshingly innovative material during the symposium (Tadić and Šoster,

The Science and Practice of Stuttering Treatment: A Symposium, First Edition. Edited by Suzana Jelčić Jakšić and Mark Onslow.

2012; Tomaiuoli et al., 2012). This was material that many of our non-European delegates had never heard before. For example, during their discussion, Tomaiuoli and colleagues proclaimed 'clients learn to express emotions through their voices and learn to modulate their voices in different ways. After that, they can say, 'Well, I gave my voice to Robert De Niro!' This is not to say that the ideas of those contributors should necessarily be endorsed because of their freshness to a non-European audience. But, to use a well-worn phrase, they might be on to something. As with all treatments considered during the symposium, we await robust clinical trials evidence of their merits, as discussed in the following text. As also considered later, there are nagging issues for treatment developers to contemplate, such as whether their developments are driven by those who stutter, by theory or merely by themselves.

There is nothing innovative with two of the symposium presenters continuing the search for the Holy Grail of a machine that drives therapy for stuttering control (Davidow, 2012) or a worn device that controls stuttering (Saltuklaroglu, 2012). However, the innovation seen at the symposium was the first presentation of what could reasonably be considered the first clinical trials of such devices: blinded assessments of their effects on stuttering during everyday conversations. Davidow outlined a successful Phase I trial of the Modification of Phonation Intervals device with five participants, and Saltuklaroglu outlined a preliminary trial of an altered auditory feedback (AAF) device. It is true that advances reported were modest, with the Phase I trial of the former device published more than a decade ago (Ingham et al., 2001). And in the latter instance it appeared – albeit debatably – that a trial of the AAF device had shown no treatment effect for stuttering control. Regardless, these two clinical trials herald what hopefully will be a future passage of such devices from the realm of pseudo-science to science (Finn et al., 2005).

The first published clinical trial of an early stuttering intervention, based on blinded assessments of everyday, post-treatment speech, was more than two decades ago (Onslow et al., 1990). During those decades, there were warning signs of staleness in this most important pursuit for our clinical researchers: to find a way to intervene early to prevent chronic stuttering. Hayhow (2012) outlined a series of clinical trials of the Lidcombe Program that, arguably, provide support for its efficacy. That being said, it is inconceivable that the first such conceptualised early stuttering intervention to be clinically trialled would be the best imaginable. A wave of fresh air blew over the delegates at Croatia as they learned that, at last, work was under way with clinical trials of two early stuttering interventions that were markedly different from the Lidcombe Program (Lasan, 2012; Trajkovski, 2012).

An innovative glitch

This symposium constituted a comprehensive sample, if not a majority, of our clinical and research authorities for this disorder at this period of our discipline's scientific history of stuttering treatment. One overriding impression from the event is that variants of speech restructuring treatment for chronic stuttering have persistent popularity. To reiterate, speech restructuring involves 'a new speech pattern to reduce or eliminate stuttering while sounding as natural as possible' (Onslow and Menzies, 2010). The technique emerged during the 1960s and by the mid 1980s its popularity had spread worldwide. So much so that Ingham (1984) was able to assemble a seminal account of this development under the label 'prolonged speech and its variants', and Andrews et al. (1980) reported a meta-analysis of its treatment effects, proclaiming it to be the most successful of known methods for stuttering control.

Six of seventeen symposium presentations considered treatments for children, adolescents and adults that focused primarily on this treatment (Block, 2012; Cardell, 2012; Carey and O'Brian, 2012; Cream and O'Brian, 2012; Langevin and Kully, 2012; O'Brian and Carey, 2012). They all presented supportive scientific data from clinical trials. Given that it is a robust assumption that the symposium was a reasonable sample of world authorities, it is intriguing to contemplate that more than one-third of its contents dealt with a treatment that can no longer be considered innovative. In fact, three of the six presentations (Block, 2012; Cardell, 2012; Langevin and Kully, 2012) described a treatment conducted with a multiday intensive format that was designed during the 1960s (see Ingham, 1984).

Perhaps all this can be explained because our clinical science in support of such a treatment is robust, and we have found an indisputable best treatment for stuttering control. However, as considered later, to say the least, such an assertion about our science could well be challenged.

Health economics of intensive speech restructuring treatment

The viability of such treatment formats might not be so suitable for a modern speech pathology world influenced by health economics. Indeed, subsequent to its apogee during the 1980s, a decline in the popularity and availability of intensive speech restructuring treatment can be attributed to economic factors. One example is the closure in 1995 of a prominent Australian programme (Andrews, personal communication, 8 March 2003; Neilson and Andrews, 1993) that arguably was the most comprehensively researched internationally (Andrews and Feyer, 1985). The author is aware also of three similar Australian intensive speech restructuring treatment facilities that were closed, presumably for similar reasons. Australia's prominent intensive speech restructuring treatment for children (Druce et al., 1997) met a similar fate.

On economic grounds, there is a challenging aspect to some of the supportive scientific data presented during the symposium about multiday intensive treatment formats. The 3-week residential treatment described by Langevin and Kully (2012) seems to be four times more resource intensive than the 5-day non-residential format described by Block (2012). Yet, at least for the short to medium term, the two programmes appear to yield similar results. Block reported stuttering rates of around 2.0 %SS at 3.5-5 years post-treatment. Langevin and Kully did not present data for an equivalent post-treatment period, however, another report of the ISTAR programme (Langevin et al.,

2010) provides a mean 4-year post-treatment stuttering rate of 3.8 %SS. Both those results constitute around 80% stuttering reduction, despite the difference between the two in resource allocation. Additionally, the Camperdown Program appears to require a fraction of the resources than either of those treatments – as few as 10 clinician hours per client in telehealth format (Carey et al., 2010). Yet, at least for the short term, results appear to be similar according to data presented for intensive treatments during the symposium.

Is the popularity of speech restructuring treatment spurred by client need?

Roger Ingham (1990) introduced a simple and engaging notion to the study of stuttering. It was Baer's (1988, 1990) idea that treatments should address what clients complain about. Perhaps then, it would be tempting to assert that the persistent popularity of speech restructuring treatments reflects that the fundamental complaint of those affected is stuttered speech. Perhaps, that driving complaint is so strong that clinicians are compelled to overlook the lack of innovation with the treatment and are prepared to offer it regardless of economic considerations. Perhaps, that is why all the speech restructuring programmes described at the symposium are located at universities; the driving need for those who stutter to control that problem makes them an essential part of speech pathology preparation. And perhaps, those who stutter are so driven by the complaint of stuttered speech that they are prepared to endure the well-known problems with speech restructuring treatment: constant vigilance, unnatural-sounding speech and the ever present threat of relapse.

Could this explain the prominence of speech restructuring treatments? There are two arguments that might disrupt such a line of thought. In the first instance, it has become increasingly obvious of late that those with chronic stuttering suffer from anxiety just as much, if not more so, than they do from stuttered speech (for a review, see Iverach et al., 2011). Presumably they have done so for a long period, and have constantly informed their clinicians of that complaint. Yet, in contrast to speech restructuring, there has been virtually no evidence of clinical trials development of anxiety treatments for those who stutter (Rowley, 2012). In light of that, it would be difficult to believe that client complaint is capable of driving the clinical availability and underpinning research of any treatment for chronic stuttering.

Evidence that something apart from the needs of those who stutter drives modern treatment development and comes from the engaging observation that five of the six symposium presentations dealing with speech restructuring were by Australians. And at the risk of drawing too long a bow, the sixth was by Canadians, and the two cultures are similar in many respects, being Commonwealth countries. Inspection of Tables 1 and 2 in Onslow et al. (2008) provides evidence that this imbalance was not caused by any chance configuration of symposium delegates. Of the 15 clinical trials of speech restructuring reported there for adults and adolescents internationally, 10 were conducted in Australia and all but one of them were conducted in Australia and Canada. That cannot be coincidental. Could it be that it is communities of clinical researchers and clinicians that is driving the current popularity of speech restructuring treatment, and not the clinical needs of those who stutter? Could it be that we are serving our own needs rather than the needs of those who stutter? Could it be that the clinical community into which those who stutter are born determines what treatment they receive, rather than how their lives are affected by stuttering?

Does it matter what drives treatment development for chronic stuttering?

An inescapable observation of the symposium documentation in the foregoing pages is that those with chronic stuttering are likely to receive a different treatment according to where they live, and that the treatments offered seem more different than similar: Gradual Increase in Length and Complexity of Utterance (GILCU) or the Successful Stuttering Management Program in the United States, speech restructuring in the British Commonwealth, Conscious Synthesis of Development in Serbia and an art-mediated programme in Italy. With the exception of speech restructuring, it is difficult to identify offerings of those treatments beyond those locations. And it seems a tempting conclusion that such a situation occurs not because of what ails those who stutter but because of what the research and clinical communities at those locations think is an appropriate treatment for their clients.

There is no definitive material to be found in the foregoing pages that might indicate why these different treatments are thought by different authorities at different locations to be suitable for chronic stuttering. Underlying aetiological theory is a possibility, and symposium presenters were invited to explore the 'theoretical basis' of their treatments. Some proponents of speech restructuring were able to explain the effects of such treatments in terms of modern knowledge about the nature of stuttering and how it might be controlled (Cardell, 2012; Langevin and Kully, 2012; O'Brian and Carey, 2012). But those authors could not cite any underlying theory as the driving force of the treatment. Indeed, it would be difficult to do so considering that the essence of speech restructuring was described early in the nineteenth Century (Clark, 1964) and arguably around a century earlier (Bormann, 1969), long before the appearance of any influential theory. Three authors cited multifactorial theory as the driving force of treatments they discuss (Lasan, 2012; Tadić and Šoster, 2012; Tomaiuoli et al., 2012). However, an inevitable stumbling block for such an assertion has been spelt out clearly (Packman and Attanasio, 2004). Multifactorial theory posits a different cause for every case of stuttering, hence, it is not really an aetiological theory in the sense of offering a parsimonious explanation for the condition. Consequently, it drives a different treatment for each person who stutters.

Could there be any harm in this situation where different therapies are offered at different international locations for non-transparent reasons? Arguably not for chronic stuttering, which is generally thought to be incurable.

An ineffective treatment for an adult or adolescent who stutters ultimately is not likely to worsen the condition. Apart from delaying the arrival of a helpful treatment and prolonging human distress, the ill effects of such a scenario amount only to waste of human and economic resources.

Does it matter what drives treatment development for early stuttering?

If consideration of this matter shifts to the case of early stuttering treatment, things are much different in light of the commonly received wisdom that early stuttering during the preschool years is a far more tractable condition than later in life. Data presented by Hayhow (2012) show this to be true, with an odd ratio of 7.5 derived from meta-analysis ($N = 134$) of Lidcombe Program randomised controlled trials (RCTs) and randomised, controlled experiments. Clearly the time to act clinically and effectively is shortly after onset. At that period during life, a pointless treatment deemed appropriate for no transparent reason, spanning considerable time, could have a lasting effect on health. Put simply, an ineffective treatment during the clinical window of opportunity during the preschool years could cause rather than prevent chronic stuttering later in life.

What drives clinical presentation of early stuttering?

It seems clear that what drives clinical presentation of early stuttering is stuttered speech. What else could parents who come to clinics complain about with their children? Certainly, there is evidence that stuttering may distress preschool children and elicit negative peer reaction and poor parent coping responses (Ezrati-Vinacour et al., 2001; Langevin et al., 2009, 2010; Millard et al., 2009). Parents may report such things to clinicians. But as far as is currently known, the serious educational, occupational and social problems associated with chronic stuttering are still distant during the preschool years. The common mental health issues with chronic stuttering have not been reported for preschoolers. The problem appears in sum to be stuttering onset.

A watershed

Presenters at the symposium outlined the clinical reasoning behind their early stuttering treatments by specifying clearly that their goals are no stuttering or almost no stuttering for long periods of clinical maintenance. Such reasoning underpins the Lidcombe Program (Hayhow, 2012) and the Westmead Program (Trajkovski, 2012) trials. However such a goal might be attained, the seeking to attain it seems uncontroversial. Even Johnson's (1942) impossibly circular clinical approach that stuttering was caused by parent diagnosis was designed to stop the development of chronic stuttering.

However, the contents of the symposium have displayed what seems to be a watershed in the history of our clinical trials of early intervention. It appears that, for the first time in our history, those who conduct clinical trials are operating from divergent assumptions. The variant of multifactorial early stuttering intervention described by Lasan (2012), Parent Child Interaction therapy, specifies only that stuttering will decrease in response to treatment and that parents will show an adaptive coping response to their stuttering children. A developer of that treatment independently verifies that to be the case:

Our aim is not zero stuttering during intervention. We seek to establish a decreasing trend in stuttering, reduced parental anxiety and increased parental confidence in managing the stuttering (Onslow and Millard, 2012, p. 8).

Likewise, outlines of other multifactorial early interventions do not specify that they are intended to get rid of stuttering (Franken et al., 2005; Yaruss et al., 2006).

This watershed presents a foreseeable problem for our quest to establish comprehensive clinical trials evidence for stuttering control. According to Chambless and Hollon (1998), the surest path to such an achievement would be ultimately to determine the most efficacious treatment by comparing treatments to each other in randomised trials. But the problem is that we now have two styles of treatment that call for different outcome measures. As such, it is logically impossible to compare such treatments against each other in a clinical trial. The impending, uninterpretable literature that might ensue from such attempted comparisons is well illustrated with the Franken et al. (2005) report of a multifactorial treatment compared to the Lidcombe Program for a 12-week period, after which around half of the children would have completed the latter treatment.

Our symposium presenters have shown us three treatment styles that are contenders for early stuttering intervention. Hopefully, before long, we will have even more. Eventually, we could know across the board, which, if any, treatments have superior effects on stuttering or are more clinically efficient. We will also be able to gather knowledge about which early interventions are best suited to which children affected by stuttering, at which ages. It would be regrettable if treatments based on multifactorial therapy were to be logically excluded from that body of research.

Perhaps then, we need to include an item for urgent consideration by members of our discipline who lead stuttering treatment development. We somehow, somewhere, need to consider this issue carefully. Nippold (2011) has speculated that clinicians have given up hope of controlling the stuttering of school-age children. Are we of a similar mind with preschoolers who stutter, or does the scant evidence presented in this volume provide some hope to the contrary? Can we possibly aspire to be a discipline that finds a way to stop the development of a pernicious disorder during the preschool years, or is that too much of an aspiration? Should we be content with never having an empirically derived answer to the question 'is multifactorial treatment the best for stuttering preschoolers'? Should we be prepared to accept two independent strands of early stuttering treatment research: one designed to eliminate early stuttering and one designed to reduce its severity?

Where is the gold standard evidence?

Symposium presenters were invited to indicate the demonstrated empirical value of the treatments they discussed, and it was gratifying that all greeted the opportunity with enthusiasm. No presenter was devoid of any data that supported the merits of a treatment.

That being said, it was striking that the glittering prize of health research had not been attained by any group represented by our speakers: the meta-analysis or systematic review of Phase III RCTs support for a treatment. In fact, our field is bereft of a single example of a treatment effect found with an RCT that has been replicated by an independent group. Perhaps the nearest to that was the Lattermann et al. (2008) trial subsequent to the Jones et al. (2005) RCT of the Lidcombe Program (see Hayhow, 2012). However, although independent, the former trial cannot really be considered as a replication of Jones et al. because it presented only 16 weeks of treatment, not the entire treatment.

There are, of course, many ways to determine the merits of treatment research, but it is inescapable that a well-designed RCT, consistent with CON-SORT guidelines,[1] is the 'gold standard' of how to do so. Bothe et al. (2006) present many of the sources contending the merits of RCTs. There are those who might quibble with that contention, and indeed one of our presenters (Ryan, 2012) argued that such methods were not necessary for the GILCU treatment. Another source of dispute about a contention of the value RCT is the claimed existence of the 'Dodo effect' (Zebrowski and Arenas, 2010). This is the contention that treatment effects of various kinds have little to do with different treatments but what matters is the quality of the clinical relationship and client expectation. Millard has raised this prospect also with reference to early stuttering intervention (Onslow and Millard, 2012). Other authors (Bothe et al., 2006) have railed somewhat against the value of RCTs by arguing that single subject designs are more suited than group designs for speech-language pathology, providing tight internal experimental control and closely resembling clinical practice.

On balance, perhaps it is not going too far to submit that any argument weakening the value of the RCT as a gold standard is far from won. Certainly, no national classification system for determining the value of health research has yet been revised to take account of any such argument. These include the Oxford Centre for Evidence Based Practice (United Kingdom),[2] the National

---

[1] http://www.consort-statement.org
[2] http://www.cebm.net/index.aspx?o=1025

Cancer Institute, National Institutes of Health (United States),[3] the Joanna Briggs Institute for Evidence Based Nursing and Midwifery (Australia),[4] the National Centre for Complementary and Alternative Medicine, National Institutes of Health (United States)[5] and the National Health and Medical Research Council (Australia) (National Health and Medical Research Council, 1999).

The limitations of non-randomised evidence

There is no doubt that non-randomised Phase I and Phase II clinical trials are necessary, intermediate steps to obtaining best evidence RCTs. But they have their limitations. Trajkovski (2012), for example, presents a single subject experiment with three children as Phase I evidence for the Westmead Program. Although Bothe et al. (2006) are correct in their argument that such designs have tight internal validity, their small participant numbers do not provide clinicians what they really need to know; what is the likely treatment effect size for the population of those who stutter that they will encounter in daily clinical practice? Even non-randomised Phase II trials comprising substantial participant numbers (Block, 2012; Cardell, 2012; Langevin and Kully, 2012; Trajkovski, 2012) have limitations in providing a trustworthy estimate of treatment effect size. Those limitations arise from biases that influence effect size estimates, leading to overestimates of what the true effect size of a treatment might be (Kunz and Oxman, 1998). Obvious sources of such bias are regression to the mean, placebo effects and, in the case of young participants, natural recovery. Allocation bias is a particular concern with non-randomised clinical trials. Allocation bias occurs where the participant and the researcher are the sole deciders of whether a participant receives the experimental treatment, rather than an independent randomisation process that occurs with an RCT. With clinical trials conducted in standard service provision facilities, as is the case with many of the trials reported by our presenters, allocation bias favours participants who are prone to be successful with the treatment in question, and exclude from it those who are prone to be unsuccessful.

The reality of this issue can be seen by comparing the results of non-randomised Phase II trials and RCTs presented in this volume. It seems reasonable to state that the Phase II reports invariably show a better treatment effect than the RCT reports that compare the experimental treatment with a no-treatment control. A prime example would be in Cream and O'Brian (2012), where non-randomised preliminary evidence for the effects of self-modelling is extremely encouraging but when the procedure is tested with a RCT by the same group, the evidence in support of the procedure is modest.

---

[3]http://www.cancer.gov/cancertopics/pdq/levels-evidence-adult-treatment/HealthProfessional/page1
[4]http://www.joannabriggs.edu.au/
[5]http://nccam.nih.gov/research/clinicaltrials/factsheet/

In short, among the conclusions to this volume must be that there is no compelling evidence based on replicated, well-conducted RCTs that any of the treatments considered here are efficacious and that their effect sizes are well established. Put simply, perhaps even bluntly, the presenters of this volume are in no position to make statements – positive or otherwise – to the clinical communities they lead about the value of treatments. At best, the collective weight of this volume could amount only to a cautiously positive statement that clinical trials have shown preliminary promise for some treatments.

How serious is the problem?

Lest it is not fully clear, the gravity of this situation can be conveyed in various ways. To return to the issue of the prominence of speech restructuring treatments, more than 30 years ago, Andrews et al. (1980) reported a meta-analysis report of this treatment. Referring to speech restructuring variants, they concluded that 'speech and gentle onset techniques' (p. 303) provided superior benefits to other treatments. Today, three decades later, with no RCTs to inform us, we seem to be in fairly much the same position. We certainly are light years away from having what Chambless and Hollon (1998) argue is real clinical trials advancement: the experimental comparison of treatments against each other to know which is better.[6]

Quantifying the problem

Another insight into the seriousness of this situation can be obtained with reference to the Institute for Scientific Information Web of Science database. Searches of other non-medical health sciences that deal with a specific disorder – analogues to our own field of speech-language pathology dealing with stuttering – are presented in Table 18.1. Although such bibliometric comparisons have their notorious shortcomings, the results of Table 18.1 are nonetheless illuminating. Considering the peer-reviewed journal articles that appear in that database, the discipline of speech pathology has published more papers about stuttering than the discipline of physiotherapy has about back pain and the discipline of occupational therapy has about falls. In contrast, and perhaps most revealing, the proportions of that peer-reviewed output for stuttering that are RCTs are around a quarter of a percent, but the proportions for back pain and falls approach 10%. In short, compared to cognate disciplines and some disorders for which they are responsible, our discipline seems to publish much more about stuttering but proportionally much less of those publications are RCTs.

---

[6]The body of clinical trials literature in this volume tangentially skirts this issue on one occasion, which is the comparison not of two different speech restructuring techniques, but of different ways of presenting them to clients (Carey et al., 2010).

Table 18.1 Search of the Institute of Science Web of Science data base showing number of publications, RCTs and percentage of publications that are RCTs for the disorders of stuttering, back pain and falls. (Date of search, October 2011.)

	Disorder	Topic search criteria	Publications	RCTs	Percentage RCTs
Speech pathology	Stuttering	Stuttering *and* speech	1546	4[a]	0.26
Physiotherapy	Back pain	Physiotherapy *and* back pain	950	88	9.3
Occupational therapy	Falls	Occupational therapy *and* falls	108	9	8.3

RCT, randomised controlled trial.
[a]This search listed the Jones et al. (2008) follow-up to the Jones et al. (2005) RCT, so the former was deleted from the search results.

What caused the problem?

So what might explain this unusual state of affairs with our discipline's efforts with stuttering treatments? Speech pathology, physiotherapy and occupational therapy seem to have in common that they do not have the extensive resources of the medical profession. For example, a search of the same database reveals 837 RCTs for hypertension. The disparity there is understandable. Professional preparation in the three disciplines in Table 18.1 is focused more or less exclusively on attaining a qualification for professional practice. There is little funding or infrastructure available to induce graduates to contemplate a research career in preference to a practitioner career. There is, for example, no career infrastructure in those professions that resemble the network of government funded Australian independent health and medical research institutes, at which medical graduates may train for a research career. Many of the presenters in this volume remarked that they are located at clinics and do not have funding for research. Yet in that regard, speech pathology appears to be in the same position to physiotherapy and occupational therapy. Neither can an explanation be that the speech pathology profession considers stuttering to be an inconsequential speech disorder in terms of the research attention it generates. Using the topic search terms speech therapy *or* speech pathology *or* speech-language pathology *or* speech-language therapy, a total of 5714 publications emerged. Using the data in Column Four of Table 18.1, this means that around 27% of our discipline's publications are about stuttering. Similar analyses for physiotherapy and occupational therapy reveal results of 12% and 1.6%, respectively, so uninterest in the topic cannot be an explanation. Considering that, neither can the often documented poor quality of professional clinical training with stuttering (for an overview, see Block, 2012). Regardless of that poor training, many of our graduates find their way to research locations, but not many of them conduct clinical trials. At least for now, it seems, that might be not only a bewildering fact but an inexplicable one. Certainly, it is not clear how to fix this problem, but somehow, somewhere, someone needs to put their minds to it or we may find ourselves in another 30 years from now, again, no further advanced.

So, many issues have been raised by our symposium, and it is uncertain whether they will be resolved, or even whether they will be taken account of. However, what is certain is that, regardless of whatever transpires, our discipline will be accountable for the future health care of those who stutter. After another three decades we may know wondrous scientific things about how to treat chronic stuttering. We may find a way to stop the development of early stuttering in its tracks. We may fail on both accounts. But whatever the outcome may be, our part in it is documented for an eternity as the proceedings of this symposium.

References

Andrews, G., & Feyer, A. M. (1985) Does behavior therapy still work when the experimenters depart: an analysis of a behavioral treatment program for stuttering. *Behavior Modification, 9*(4), 443-457.

Andrews, G., Guitar, B., & Howie, P. (1980) Meta-analysis of the effects of stuttering treatment. *Journal of Speech and Hearing Disorders, 45,* 287-307.

Baer, D. (1988) If you know why you're changing a behavior, you'll know when you've changed it enough. *Behavioral Assessment, 10,* 219-223.

Baer, D. (1990) The critical issue in treatment efficacy is knowing why treatment was applied: a student's response to Roger Ingham. In: L. Olswang, C. Thompson, S. Warren & N. Minghetti (Eds.), *Treatment Efficacy Research in Communication Disorders* (pp. 31-39). Rockville, MD: American Speech-Language-Hearing Foundation.

Block, S. (2012) Student-delivered treatment for stuttering: multiday intensive speech restructuring. In: S. Jelcic Jaksic & M. Onslow (Eds.), *The Science and Practice of Stuttering Treatment* (Chapter 7, pp. 87-98). Oxford: John Wiley & Sons.

Bormann, E. G. (1969) Ephphatha, or some advice to stammerers. *Journal of Speech and Hearing Research, 12*(3), 453-461.

Bothe, A. K., Davidow, J. H., Bramlett, R. E., Franic, D. M., & Ingham, R. J. (2006) Stuttering treatment research 1970-2005: II. Systematic review incorporating trial quality assessment of pharmacological approaches. *American Journal of Speech-Language Pathology, 15,* 342-352.

Cardell, L. (2012) Intensive speech restructuring treatment for school-age children. In: S. Jelcic Jaksic & M. Onslow (Eds.), *The Science and Practice of Stuttering Treatment* (Chapter 6, pp. 71-86). Oxford: John Wiley & Sons.

Carey, B., & O'Brian, S. (2012) Telehealth treatments for stuttering control. In: S. Jelcic Jaksic & M. Onslow (Eds.), *The Science and Practice of Stuttering Treatment* (Chapter 10, pp. 131-146). Oxford: John Wiley & Sons.

Carey, B., O'Brian, S., Onslow, M., Block, S., Packman, A., & Jones, M. (2010) A randomised controlled non-inferiority trial of a telehealth treatment for chronic stuttering: the Camperdown Program. *International Journal of Language and Communication Disorders, 45,* 108-120.

Chambless, D. L., & Hollon, S. D. (1998) Defining empirically supported therapies. *Journal of Consulting and Clinical Psychology, 66,* 7-18.

Clark, R. M. (1964). Our enterprising predecessors and Charles Sydney Bluemel. *ASHA, 6*(4), 107-114.

CONSORT: transparent reporting of clinical trials. Retrieved from http://www.consort-statement.org/

Cream, A., & O'Brian, S. (2012) Self-modeling for chronic stuttering. In: S. Jelcic Jaksic & M. Onslow (Eds.), *The Science and Practice of Stuttering Treatment* (Chapter 12, pp. 159-170). Oxford: John Wiley & Sons.

Davidow, J. (2012) Modifying phonation interval stuttering treatment program. In: S. Jelcic Jaksic & M. Onslow (Eds.), *The Science and Practice of Stuttering Treatment* (Chapter 1, pp. 1-14). Oxford: John Wiley & Sons.

Druce, T., Debney, S., & Byrt, T. (1997) Evaluation of an intensive treatment program for stuttering in young children. *Journal of Fluency Disorders, 22,* 169-186.

Ezrati-Vinacour, R., Platzky, R., & Yairi, E. (2001) The young child's awareness of stuttering-like disfluency. *Journal of Speech Language and Hearing Research, 44,* 368-380.

Finn, P., Bothe, A. K., & Bramlett, R. E. (2005) Science and pseudoscience in communication disorders: criteria and applications. *American Journal of Speech-Language Pathology, 14,* 172-186.

Franken, M. C., Kielstra-Van der Schalk, C. J., & Boelens, H. (2005) Experimental treatment of early stuttering: a preliminary study. *Journal of Fluency Disorders, 30,* 189-199.

Hayhow, R. (2012) The Lidcombe Program. In: S. Jelcic Jaksic & M. Onslow (Eds.), *The Science and Practice of Stuttering Treatment* (Chapter 4, pp. 43-56). Oxford: John Wiley & Sons.

Ingham, R. J. (1984) *Stuttering and Behavior Therapy: Current Status and Experimental Foundations.* San Diego, CA: College-Hill Press.

Ingham, R. (1990) Theoretical, methodological, and ethical issues in treatment efficacy research: stuttering therapy as a case study. In: L. Olswang, C. Thompson, S. Warren & N. Minghetti (Eds.), *Treatment Efficacy Research in Communication Disorders* (pp. 15-29). Rockville, MD: American Speech-Language-Hearing Association.

Ingham, R. J., Kilgo, M., Ingham, J. C., Moglia, R., Belknap, H., & Sanchez, T. (2001) Evaluation of a stuttering treatment based on reduction of short phonation intervals. *Journal of Speech Language and Hearing Research, 44,* 1229-1244.

Iverach, L., Menzies, R., O'Brian, S., Packman, A., & Onslow, M. (2011) Anxiety and stuttering: Continuing to explore a complex relationship. *American Journal of Speech Language Pathology, 20,* 221-232.

Johnson, W. (1942) A study of the onset and development of stuttering. *Journal of Speech and Hearing Disorders, 7,* 251-257.

Jones, M., Onslow, M., Packman, A., Williams, S., Ormond, T., Schwarz, I., & Gebski, V. (2005) Randomised controlled trial of the Lidcombe programme of early stuttering intervention. *British Medical Journal, 331,* 659-661.

Jones, M., Onslow, M., Packman, A., O'Brian, S., Hearne, A., Williams, S., & Schwarz, I. (2008) Extended follow-up of a randomised controlled trial of the Lidcombe Program of Early Stuttering Intervention. *International Journal of Language and Communication Disorders, 43,* 649-661.

Kunz, R., & Oxman, A. (1998) The unpredictability paradox: review of empirical comparisons of randomised and non-randomised clinical trials. *British Medical Journal, 317,* 1185-1190.

Langevin, M., & Kully, D. (2012) The comprehensive stuttering program and its evidence base. In: S. Jelcic Jaksic & M. Onslow (Eds.), *The Science and Practice of Stuttering Treatment* (Chapter 9, pp. 115-130). Oxford: John Wiley & Sons.

Langevin, M., Packman, A., & Onslow, M. (2009) Peer responses to stuttered utterances. *American Journal of Speech Language Pathology, 18*, 264-276.

Langevin, M., Packman, A., & Onslow, M. (2010) Parent perceptions of the impact of stuttering on their preschoolers and themselves. *Journal of Communication Disorders, 43*, 407-423.

Langevin, M., Kully, D., Teshima, S., Hagler, P., & Narasimha Prasad, N. G. (2010) Five-year longitudinal treatment outcomes of the ISTAR Comprehensive Stuttering Program. *Journal of Fluency Disorders, 35*, 123-40.

Lasan, M. (2012) Multifactorial treatment for preschool children. In: S. Jelcic Jaksic & M. Onslow (Eds.), *The Science and Practice of Stuttering Treatment* (Chapter 13, pp. 171-182). Oxford: John Wiley & Sons.

Lattermann, C., Euler, H. A., & Neumann, K. (2008) A randomized control trial to investigate the impact of the Lidcombe Program on early stuttering in German-speaking preschoolers. *Journal of Fluency Disorders, 33*, 52-65.

Millard, S. K., Edwards, S., & Cook, F. M. (2009) Parent-child interaction therapy: adding to the evidence. *International Journal of Speech- Language Pathology, 11*, 61-76.

National Cancer Institute Levels of Evidence for Adult and Pediatric Cancer Treatment Studies (PDQ®). Retrieved from http://www.cancer.gov/cancer topics/pdq/levels-evidence-adult-treatment/HealthProfessional/page1

National Health and Medical Research Council (1999) A guide to the development, implementation and evaluation of clinical practice guidelines. Commonwealth of Australia, Canberra. Retrieved from http://www.nhmrc.gov.au/_files_nhmrc/publications/attachments/cp30.pdf

Neilson, M., & Andrews, G. (1993) Intensive fluency training of chronic stutterers. In: R. Curlee (Ed.), *Stuttering and Other Disorders of Fluency* (pp. 139-165). New York: Thieme.

Nippold, M. A. (2011) Stuttering in school-age children: a call for treatment research. *Language, Speech, and Hearing Services in Schools, 42*, 99-101.

O'Brian, S., & Carey, B. (2012) The Camperdown Program. In: S. Jelcic Jaksic & M. Onslow (Eds.), *The Science and Practice of Stuttering Treatment* (Chapter 2, pp. 15-28). Oxford: John Wiley & Sons.

Onslow, M., & Menzies, R. (2010) *Speech restructuring.* Accepted entry in www.commonlanguagepsychotherapy.org

Onslow, M., & Millard, S. (2012) Palin parent child interaction and the Lidcombe Program: clarifying some issues. *Journal of Fluency Disorders, 37*, 1-8.

Onslow, M., Costa, L., & Rue, S. (1990) Direct early intervention with stuttering: some preliminary data. *Journal of Speech and Hearing Disorders, 55*, 405-416.

Onslow, M., Jones, M., O'Brian, S., Menzies, R., & Packman, A. (2008) Defining, identifying, and evaluating clinical trials of stuttering treatments: a tutorial for clinicians. *American Journal of Speech Language Pathology, 17*, 401-415.

Packman, A., & Attanasio, J. (2004) *Theoretical Issues in Stuttering.* London: Psychology Press.

Rowley, D. (2012) Cognitive behaviour therapy. In: S. Jelcic Jaksic & M. Onslow (Eds.), *The Science and Practice of Stuttering Treatment* (Chapter 14, pp. 183-194). Oxford: John Wiley & Sons.

Ryan, B. (2012) The gradual increase in length and complexity of utterance program. In: S. Jelcic Jaksic & M. Onslow (Eds.), *The Science and Practice of Stuttering Treatment* (Chapter 17, pp. 221-232). Oxford: John Wiley & Sons.

Saltuklaroglu, T. (2012) Assessment and treatment using altered auditory feedback. In: S. Jelcic Jaksic & M. Onslow (Eds.), *The Science and Practice of Stuttering Treatment* (Chapter 3, pp. 29–42). Oxford: John Wiley & Sons.

Tadić, J., & Šoster, D. (2012) Conscious synthesis of development: a holistic approach to stuttering. In: S. Jelcic Jaksic & M. Onslow (Eds.), *The Science and Practice of Stuttering Treatment* (Chapter 16, pp. 207–220). Oxford: John Wiley & Sons.

The Joanna Briggs Institute (2011) Welcome to the Joanna Briggs Institute. Retrieved from http://www.joannabriggs.edu.au/

Tomaiuoli, D., Del Gado, F., Lucchini, E., & Spinetti, M. G. (2012) A multidimensional, integrated, differentiated, art-mediated stuttering program. In: S. Jelcic Jaksic & M. Onslow (Eds.), *The Science and Practice of Stuttering Treatment* (Chapter 13, pp. 171–182). Oxford: John Wiley & Sons.

Trajkovski, N. (2012) The Westmead Program. In: S. Jelcic Jaksic & M. Onslow (Eds.), *The Science and Practice of Stuttering Treatment* (Chapter 15, pp. 195–206). Oxford: John Wiley & Sons.

Yaruss, J. S., Coleman, C., & Hammer, D. (2006) Treating preschool children who stutter: description and preliminary evaluation of a family-focused treatment approach. *Language, Speech and Hearing Services in the Schools, 37*, 118–136.

Zebrowski, P. M., & Arenas, R. M. (2010) The "Iowa Way" revisited. *Journal of Fluency Disorders, 36*, 144–157.

Index

Note: Italicised f's refer to figures.

The Science and Practice of Stuttering Treatment: A Symposium, First Edition. Edited by
Suzana Jelčić Jakšić and Mark Onslow.
© 2012 John Wiley & Sons, Ltd. Published 2012 by John Wiley & Sons, Ltd.

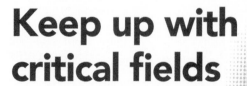
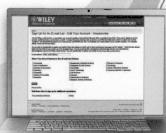
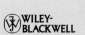